Contents

KT-528-566

Preface

First Health & Social Care provides an introduction for all students embarking on, or engaged in, a course of study in the subject. Although designed to cover the BTEC Level 2 specification, its contents overlap similar courses at this level. The students are introduced to the wide variety of jobs in the Health and Care Sectors with its workforce of over two million people. The comprehensive index and glossary allows easy access to information and also makes the book a useful reference for continuous workforce development.

First Health & Social Care is divided into ten chapters. It starts with an Introduction to the subject followed by chapters on Communication, the Needs of Individuals, Work Experience, the Diversity of Individuals, Anatomy and Physiology of the Human Body, Human Lifespan Development, Creative and Therapeutic Activities, the Health and Social Care Services, and the Impact of Diet on Health. The final chapter is devoted to Study Skills to encourage students to carry out assignments to the best of their abilities.

Tutor Resources for the book contain time-saving and practical resources for those teaching the subject. These include worksheets that progress from simple tasks to more complex exercises, case studies, blank pro-formas, activities that cover Key Skills requirements and useful website addresses.

We should like to thank all those who helped us with producing this book and, in particular, Elizabeth Ramsden (Senior Sister, Guys Hospital) and Jill Purkis (Specialist Nurse), Elizabeth Maclennan (Occupational Therapist) and Sarah Holmes (Physiotherapist) who have kindly allowed us to benefit from their extensive experience. The authors and publisher would like to acknowledge the following publication as a source for some of the medical illustrations used in this book: Cull, P. and Hague, L. (Medical College of St Bartholomew's Hospital, London) (1989) *The Sourcebook of Medical Illustration*. Carnforth: The Parthenon Publishing Group Limited.

We are indebted to our publisher, Judith Harvey, for her invaluable expert advice and friendly and immediate help whenever we have needed to contact her with our problems. Every attempt has been made to ensure accuracy, but any errors are all ours and we would be very grateful to be informed about them.

Pamela Minett
David Wayne

First
Health & Social Care

By
Pamel

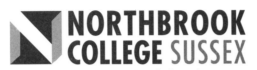

NORTHBROOK COLLEGE SUSSEX
Further, Higher and Adult Education

Library and Information Services

BW

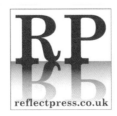

reflectpress.co.uk

Reflect Press Ltd

www.reflectpress.co.uk

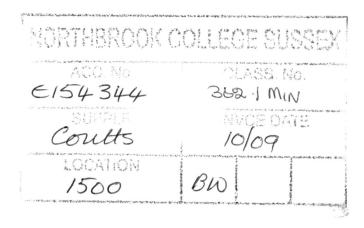
First published in 2009

ISBN: 978 1 906052 17 1

British Library Cataloguing in Publication Data
A catalogue record for this book is available from the British Library

Production project management by Deer Park Productions
Graphics by Graham Hiles (Media Services)
Illustrations by Greg Lindsay-Smith (One Vision Illustration)
Typeset by Kestrel Data, Exeter
Cover design and medical illustrations by OXMED
Printed and bound by Bell & Bain Ltd, Glasgow
Distributed by BEBC, Albion Close, Parkstone, Poole, Dorset BH12 3LL

Published by Reflect Press Ltd
11 Attwyll Avenue
Exeter
Devon, EX2 5HN
UK
01392 204400

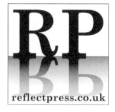

reflectpress.co.uk

Reflect Press Ltd
www.reflectpress.co.uk

First Health & Social Care

Introduction

'First Health & Social Care' is designed for students intending to enter the health and social care workforce or as a basis for higher qualifications in the subject.

The **contents** provide a framework of knowlege on which you can build as your studies progress.

The **questions** encourage your understanding of the text.

The **activities** aim to broaden your knowledge, to reinforce and extend your learning experience, and to assist you in the attainment of qualifications.

Health and Social Care

Health and Social Care is the study of the care services that we all need at different times in our lives. The **Health Care services** provide for our mental and physical well-being. The **Social Care services** look after our general welfare. When required, they work together in partnership as, for example, in the **Early Years services** that provide health care, social care and education to children aged 0–8 years.

Terms used by the care services

- **Service providers** are the organisations that provide caring services such as hospitals, health centres, social services and services that support children and their families.
- **Care professionals** are people who have been specially trained and have gained the relevant qualifications, for example doctors, nurses and social workers. Care professionals are supported by many others who work in the caring services such as medical secretaries and receptionists.
- **Carers** look after those people who cannot look after themselves, for example support workers, care assistants and home carers.
- **Service users** are patients, clients or customers who use the health and social care services. Generally, people who use health care services are called **patients**; those using the social care services are called **clients** or **customers**.

Aims of care work

The central purpose of all the Health and Social Care services for patients and clients is to:

- improve their quality of life;
- enable them to take control of their own lives;
- help them maintain or establish links with family, friends and society;
- respect their choices, even if they conflict with given advice;
- to treat everyone equally whatever their race or beliefs.

Statements illustrating the five aims of care work

A   Care services available to everyone in need.

B   Support for people with disabilities to enable them to live independently.

C   Medical advice was not followed, but care continued to be provided.

D   Knee and hip operations that enable people to walk without pain.

E   Volunteer drivers who take disabled people to day care centres and outings.

Activity

Working with a partner or in a small group make a list of occasions when you, your families or friends have used the:
i   Health Care services.
ii   Social Care services.
(➲ Making notes page 242.)

1. a Name three types of care services and their functions.
   b Who are: i service providers, ii service users?
   c In the caring services, who are called: i care professionals, ii carers, iii patients, iv customers or clients?
   d List the five aims of care work and give an appropriate example from the box above.
(➲ Answering questions page 241.)

Working in the caring services

Health and care workers formed the largest occupational group in England and Wales in 2001. Two and a half million people were employed in the various health and social care services. This included both the public and private sectors, but not the unpaid voluntary carers.

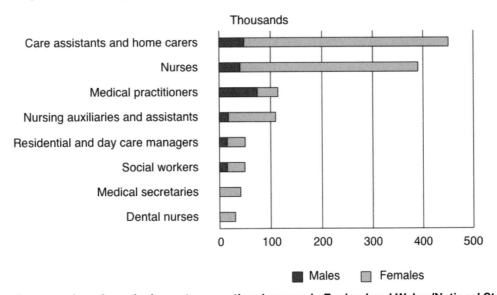

Health and care workers form the largest occupational groups in England and Wales (National Statistics)

Skills for caring

Working in health and social care services is all about working with people. In addition to any specialist qualifications required for the job, the other skills needed include the ability to:

- communicate easily with patients, clients and colleagues;
- listen to what they have to say;
- treat them with respect;
- value them as individuals;
- respect their rights and beliefs.

2. a How many people were employed in the health and care services in England and Wales in 2001?
  b From the chart above, sort the groups into
    i health care (5 groups),
    ii social care (3 groups).
  c Which of the groups:
    i is the largest group in the chart,
    ii has more men than women,
    iii has no men?
  d Name five caring skills.

Activity

For every thousand people in England and Wales there are:
  86 care assistants and home carers
  75 nurses
  22 doctors
  5 midwives
  4 dentists
Use this information to produce a pie chart for 'Health and Care Workers in England and Wales'.

Health care, social care and early years services

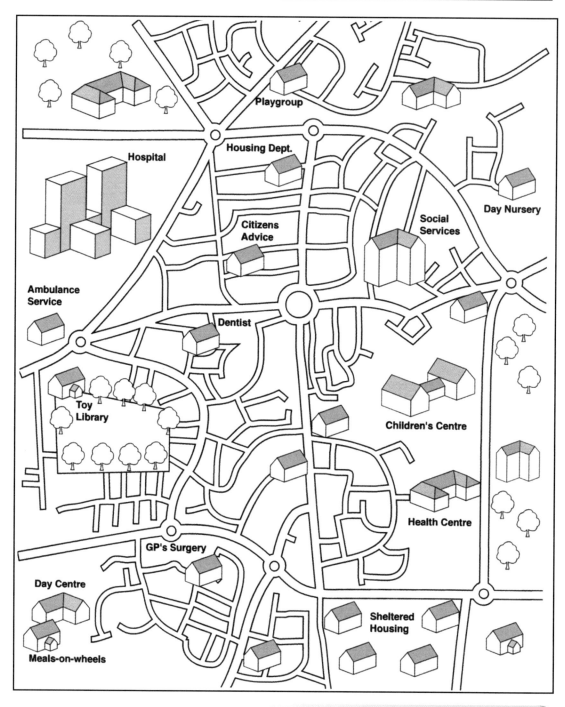

1. Copy the table below then place the caring services named on the plan above into the appropriate column (5 in each group).

Activity

On a street map of your nearest town, mark in the services for Health Care, Social Care and Early Years. Colour code and make a key.

	Health Care	Social Care	Early Years
1			
2			
3			
4			
5			

Chapter 1
Communication and Individual Rights

This chapter covers:

- The different forms of communication, promotion of effective communication, communication skills and the communication cycle.

- Barriers to effective communication and ways of overcoming them.

- Factors that create diversity in society and those that promote equality.

- Care values, the Care Value Base, and the rights and responsibilities of individuals and workers in society.

Communication

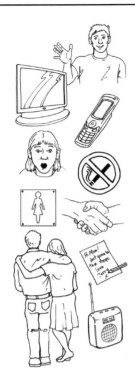

Communication is the exchange of information between individuals, groups and organisations and is an essential part of the work of the health and social care sectors. Good communication skills are needed in order to develop relationships with patients, clients and their relatives, and also with colleagues, managers and other professionals.

Formal communications are usually written communications because the information they contain needs to be recorded so that it can be referred to again. They include letters, emails, reports and instructions. **Informal communications** are usually light-hearted and friendly. They include notes, text messages, phone calls, casual greetings, and also occur when people are just chatting together. **Verbal communication** uses words in speech or writing. **Non-verbal communication** is by body language, symbols, signs and pictures.

Speech

The voice can be used to greet people, ask and answer questions, give instructions and make telephone calls. Information is conveyed both by the words used and the tone of voice (normal, angry, sharp, weak, excited).

Writing and pictures

These can be in the form of:

- letters, notes, reports, posters, emails, texting;
- signs for directions, road names and hazard signs;
- symbols – male and female toilets, a white stick;
- images (pictures) such as photographs, drawings.

Body language

Body language is communication by movements or position of the body. Information can be conveyed by:

- the head – a nod, shake, held high, drooping;
- eyes – eye contact, rolling the eyes, raising eyebrows, weeping;
- facial expressions – smile, frown, bored, interested;
- posture – sitting or standing upright, slouching, dejected;
- walking – slowly, quickly, limping, stomping away in anger;
- arms – folded, hugging, pushing, waving;
- hands – touching, pointing, clenching the fist.

Multi-media communication

Radio, computers, mobile phones, iPods, videos, TV, CDs and DVDs involve both verbal and non-verbal means of communication.

1. a What is communication?

b Explain the difference between:
  i formal and informal communication
  ii verbal and non-verbal communication.

c In what ways can writing and pictures be used to communicate?

d Which parts of the body may be involved in body language?

e What technology is used in multimedia communication?

f Identify the different forms of communication shown in the drawings above.

Activity

Look around you to find examples of different ways of communicating. Using the headings on this page, make notes of what you observe. (➲ Making notes page 242.)

Effective communication

Communication is effective when information (facts, feelings, news, etc.) is exchanged and understood by the people it concerns. People communicate most effectively when they:

- **are feeling at ease**;
- **are sincere** – this means being open and honest, and consistent in their approach;
- **are able to empathise** – empathy is the ability to understand another person's feelings by putting yourself in their place or by having had a similar experience;
- **give verbal and non-verbal messages that support each other** – if there is a mismatch between verbal and non-verbal messages, the receiver will believe the non-verbal message;
- **have good listening skills** – these are needed for **active listening** – the ability to listen in a way that shows interest, understanding and respect for what the other person is saying.

2. a i What is meant by effective communication?
  ii what are the benefits?
 b When do people communicate most effectively?
 c What is active listening?
 d Describe six listening skills.
 e Give three benefits of listening skills.

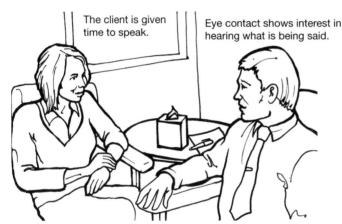

The client is given time to speak.

Eye contact shows interest in hearing what is being said.

The expression on the carer's face indicates that what the client is saying is important.

Wait for a gap in the conversation before speaking and do not interrupt.

Important points made by the client, and repeated by the carer, shows that the carer has been listening.

Occasional silences give time to reflect on what is being said.

Occasionally summing up what has been said reinforces the points being made.

Listening skills shown by a carer when talking with a client

Benefits of effective communication

When communication is effective:

- **carers** are more able to give and receive information, and understand the clients' needs;
- **service users** feel respected as individuals, find it easier to discuss their situation openly and are more likely to receive a better outcome;
- **colleagues** are kept informed.

Stressful communication

This can result from:

- **inappropriate touch** such as unwanted hugging, pushing or fondling;
- **sexual remarks** and jokes that are out of place;
- **criticism** of appearance or behaviour intended to hurt.

Activity

Watch an extract from a video/DVD to look for examples of the ways in which information is exchanged. Record them under the headings:
- Verbal communication
- Non-verbal communication
- Informal communication
- Multimedia communication.
(➲ Making notes page 242.)

Communication skills (interpersonal skills)

Care workers who have good communication skills:

- show respect for their service users;
- use friendly body language and tone of voice;
- choose a private place to discuss confidential matters;
- listen carefully to what the service user is saying;
- talk to people in a way that they can understand;
- give the service users enough time to express opinions;
- have a non-judgemental attitude;
- understand and value cultural differences;
- provide relevant and helpful information.

Giving information and instructions

Information and instructions can be difficult to remember at the best of times, but more so when the client is too nervous to concentrate, cannot understand them, or they are too complicated to remember. Therefore, when giving information and instructions to clients and patients, care workers should:

- do so in a calm manner;
- make sure they are understood by asking the person to repeat the instructions;
- provide opportunities to ask questions about them;
- help the client remember by writing them out simply.

Activity

a With a fellow student, role-play a scene similar to the one above where you take the part of a receptionist with good communication skills.

b Ask for feedback from your group and assess your performance against the good communication skills and the way to give information and instructions discussed here.

c Identify ways in which your communication skills might have been improved.

(➲ Role-play page 244.)

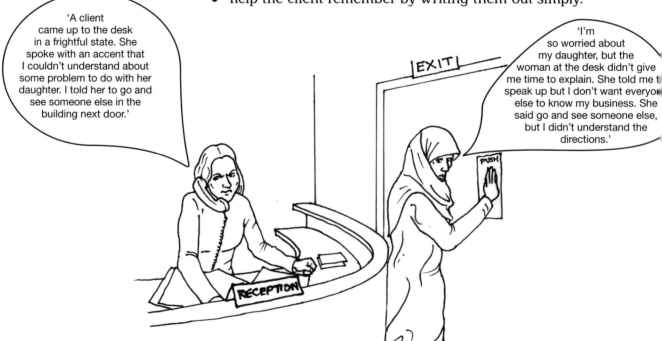

'A client came up to the desk in a frightful state. She spoke with an accent that I couldn't understand about some problem to do with her daughter. I told her to go and see someone else in the building next door.'

'I'm so worried about my daughter, but the woman at the desk didn't give me time to explain. She told me t speak up but I don't want everyo else to know my business. She said go and see someone else, but I didn't understand the directions.'

EXIT

PUSH

RECEPTION

3. a i What are interpersonal skills?
   ii Give four examples of when they are needed.
   b Name eight communication skills that the receptionist above lacked.
   c When are instructions more difficult to remember?
   d Describe a way to give instructions.

One-to-one communications

These are usually about personal matters and are often private. They require good communication skills because what a carer says and how it is said can be comforting and helpful to the client or patient, or it can cause confusion and anxiety. Giving clear instructions or information can prevent misunderstandings and also save time.

Group communications

Communicating with others takes place at meetings. It is more effective if everyone present:

- listens carefully to the speaker without interrupting;
- takes turns in expressing their views;
- respects other people's points of view;
- does not have a private conversation;
- does not make unpleasant or irrelevant remarks.

(See also 'Group discussions' ➲ page 243.)

The communication cycle

A **communication cycle** is the pathway that a message takes as it passes from a person to one or more people. It will have a sender, a means of communication, a receiver and a response.

Activities

1. Send a message to a friend.
   a Decide the purpose of the message, the form it will take and how it will be delivered.
   b Find out from your friend: how the message was received, whether it was understood, what the response was.
   c Record the message in a communication cycle.
2. Take part in a group discussion to plan a fund-raising event for a particular charity.
(➲ Group discussions page 243.)

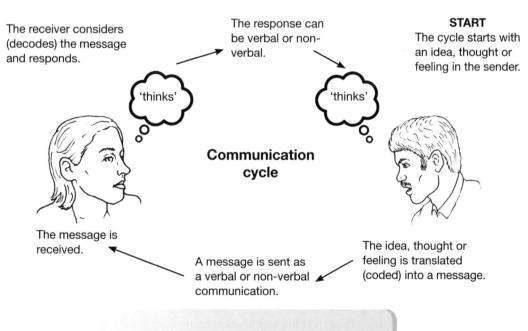

The receiver considers (decodes) the message and responds.

The response can be verbal or non-verbal.

START
The cycle starts with an idea, thought or feeling in the sender.

'thinks'

'thinks'

Communication cycle

The message is received.

A message is sent as a verbal or non-verbal communication.

The idea, thought or feeling is translated (coded) into a message.

4. a When a carer communicates with a client, give two reasons why good communication skills are essential.
   b How can speakers at group meetings communicate effectively?
   c What is a communication cycle?

Barriers to communication

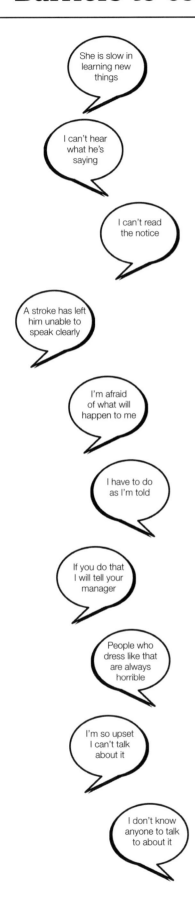

When communication is difficult or impossible between people it can be due to a barrier that exists between them.

Physical barriers are due to physical and sensory disabilities such as:

- a learning disability;
- deafness;
- poor eyesight;
- a speech defect.

Emotional barriers are due to feelings of:

- fear;
- aggression;
- threat;
- prejudice;
- distress;
- loneliness.

Language barriers prevent people from communicating easily with each other. The cause may be:

accent – the way words are pronounced by people who come from a particular place. For example, speaking English with a regional or foreign accent.

dialect – is the term used to describe differences in the way words are used in different areas. Dialects belong to different places and are usually spoken with the accent of the same area.

slang – very informal words used by a set of people.

jargon – specialised words used by a particular set of people, often as part of their job.

acronyms and abbreviations – words made from the first letters of other words such as NMC (Nursing and Midwifery Council) and GSCC (General Social Care Council).

a foreign language being spoken.

a different sense of humour – remarks intended to be funny that are misinterpreted.

talking to quickly for the listener to understand.

Environmental barriers are caused by:

- noise;
- lack of privacy.

1. **a** Select a speech bubble that applies to each of the four physical barriers.
   b Select a speech bubble that applies to each of the six emotional barriers.
   c Give the meaning of: **i** accent; **ii** dialect; **iii** slang; **iv** jargon; **v** acronym.
   d Suggest ways of removing environmental barriers to communication.

Activity

Listen to the way that different people speak and find examples of accent, dialect, slang and jargon.

Barriers in care settings

In health and care settings, barriers to communication can be due to both service users and their carers.

Service users

Clients and patients find it more difficult or impossible to communicate when they:

- are confused by unfamiliar surroundings;
- feel intimidated by people in authority;
- are afraid of what might happen;
- are unable to understand what is being said to them;
- are too ill to cooperate;
- are too young to know what is happening;
- have speech difficulties, poor eyesight or are hard of hearing;
- are in a noisy environment or lack privacy.

Behaviour of carers

There are a number of ways in which the behaviour of carers can create barriers between them and their clients or patients.

In conversation – when the carer does not listen to what the client is saying, does not give the client enough time to explain, or shows other evidence that they are not interested.

When the carer controls the client by making all the decisions – what the client should wear, where to sit and the choice of meals.

When the carer shouts at clients, or calls them names such as stupid or dirty, laughs at them or tells stories about them that cause distress.

When the carer uses negative body language such as not looking at the client, or rolling the eyes and shrugging the shoulders, or by having a severe expression on the face that forbids conversation.

When the carer shows lack of sensitivity during practical care of the client, for example rushing the client during bathing, not combing the hair, or not attending to personal needs with gentleness.

When there is a lack of resources for those with impaired hearing or sight, or those with speech or learning disabilities.

2. a When may communication barriers be due to service users?
   b Under the heading 'Preventing barriers to communication', suggest ways of preventing each of the barriers caused by the behaviour of carers.

Activity

a Explain what is meant by effective communication.
b Identify barriers that could prevent effective communication.
c Suggest ways in which they could be overcome.

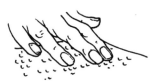

A **bliss board** is an electronic board for people who cannot speak but can point to the appropriate picture or words.

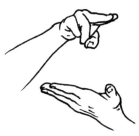

Braille is a system of raised dots used by blind people for reading and writing.

Sign language is a method of communication that uses the hands to convey messages. It enables people who are deaf to communicate with others.

Overcoming barriers to communication

When service users find it difficult to communicate, they can be helped in a number of ways.

Encouragement from carers

Carers encourage service users to communicate when they:

- make eye contact, have a friendly attitude and a warm smile;
- find a suitable place for conversation that is quiet and private;
- show that they are listening to what is being said;
- have **empathy** – the ability to understand another person's feelings;
- use sketches, pictures and pamphlets to help with explanations.

Using human aids

These are people who assist with communication and they can be:

- **signers** who use their hands to convey messages to and from people who are deaf;
- **interpreters** who convert speech from one language to another;
- **translators** who convert documents from one language to another;
- **advocates** who speak or act on behalf of a patient or client.

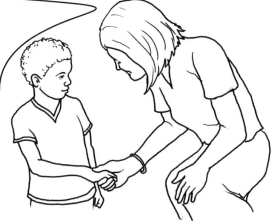

Hello John, I'm Julie your social worker. Is it alright if I ask you some questions? I've brought some pictures to help explain things to you.

Activity

In your own words, explain how communication skills can be used in a health or social care setting to assist effective communication.

3. a Name three ways in which Julie is encouraging her client to communicate.
   b What is empathy?
   c When there is a communication difficulty, describe four types of people who may be called upon to help.
   d When may the following be useful?
   i a bliss board; ii Braille; iii sign language.

Culture and communication

Culture relates to the way of life of a group of people including their customs and values. Communication is more difficult between people of different cultural backgrounds because behaviour that is usual in one culture can cause offence or be misleading to other cultures. Some examples are given below.

Names People vary in how they wish to be addressed. Some patients or clients are happy when carers call them by their first name, others find this offensive, especially when their first name is used by strangers and people much younger. They may prefer to be known as Mr . . . or Mrs . . . The best practice for carers is to ask their clients and patients how they wish to be addressed.

Greeting In many cultures it is common for people to shake hands when first introduced but, in some cultures, women do not shake hands with men. A nod of the head and a smile is not likely to offend.

Close contact Physical contact such as touching, hugging and cheek kissing may not be acceptable and is best avoided.

Eye contact It is usual to look at people when speaking to them, but in some cultures maintaining eye contact is regarded as being too controlling or confident, and in others looking away can be seen as being sly or rude.

Sense of humour Making jokes is best avoided by carers because things that are regarded as funny by the care worker may be offensive to others.

Expressing feelings People from some cultural backgrounds are reluctant to reveal their feelings or attitudes or to discuss private matters with strangers.

Gender In some cultures, privacy is very important, and treatment by someone of the same gender is preferred. Female patients may also be reluctant to remove clothing.

4. **a** Describe the conditions that enable people to communicate effectively.
   b In what ways does effective communication benefit:
   i carers,
   ii clients?
   c Give some examples of messages that can be misunderstood because of cultural differences.

Activity

a Take part in a discussion on 'The need for good communication skills by care workers when dealing with service users of other cultures'.
b Ask for feedback on your part in the discussion and assess your performance against the good communication skills and the way to give instructions and information listed on page 8.

Diversity and equality in society

A **society** is a group of individuals living together in an organised way with common characteristics such as nationality, race or religion. **Diversity** refers to the differences (diversity) between individuals in a society. Each person has their own genetic make-up and personal life-history, hopes, fears, expectations and many other factors. **Equality** means giving equal treatment to people in similar situations so that the same opportunities exist for everyone. Diversity and equality are affected by both social and political factors.

Social factors

Social factors that contribute to diversity include: culture, ethnicity, gender, sexuality, age, family structure, income, social class and geographical location.

Culture

All societies have their own culture and way of life, including the aspects given below.

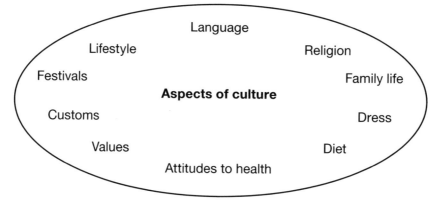

Language
Lifestyle
Religion
Festivals
Family life
Aspects of culture
Customs
Dress
Values
Diet
Attitudes to health

Ethnicity

An **ethnic group** is a group of people who share the same racial origins and cultural traditions. They may have distinctive physical features or a common language or religion. There are many ethnic groups from all parts of the world living in the UK.

A **multicultural society** is one containing different ethnic groups each with its own cultural traditions.

Activity

Compare your own culture with that of someone of a different culture. This person may be someone you know personally, or a character from a television series. Present your work in two columns under the heading 'Comparison of two cultures'.

1. **a** What is a society?
   b What is the meaning of:
   i diversity; **ii** equality.
   c Name seven social factors which make people different from each other.
   d Name 10 aspects of culture.
   e Explain the difference between an ethnic group and a multicultural society.

Gender

There are two genders – male and female. Certain behaviours, attitudes and skills may be considered more appropriate for one gender than the other. This applies more to some cultures and religions than others.

Sexuality (sexual orientation)

Most people are **heterosexual** – sexually attracted to the opposite sex. Some are **homosexual** ('gay') – sexually attracted to the same sex; women homosexuals are called **lesbians. Bisexual** means being sexually attracted to both sexes. **Homophobia** is the intense dislike of homosexual people. (➲ page 70.)

Age

Life span can last for a 100 years or more. From birth onwards changes take place as an individual grows, develops and ages, with different abilities and needs at various stages. (➲ Chapter 6.)

Family structure

There are different types of family:

- **nuclear families** consist of a man and a woman and their dependent children who all live together;
- **extended families** are large family groups that include grandparents, parents, children, aunts, uncles and cousins;
- **step families** (reconstituted families) are those with a child (or children) who is the natural child of one of the partners in a marriage or partnership but not of both;
- **lone parent (one-parent) families** consist of one adult living with children. This is caused by divorce, death, partnership break-up, or no partner from the beginning;
- **single-parent families** have one adult who has chosen to remain single while rearing dependent children;
- **adoptive families** have children who are the legal responsibility of the adults but not born to them;
- **foster families** are families temporarily caring for children who are not related to them;
- **gender families** are those where a couple of the same gender have chosen to adopt one or more children.

2. **a i** Name the two gender groups.
   ii What is a gender family?
   b Explain the difference between:
   i heterosexual and bisexual,
   ii homosexual and homophobia.
   c Explain the difference between:
   i nuclear and extended families,
   ii lone parents and single parents,
   iii adoptive and foster families.
   d What is a step family?

Geographical location

The place where a person grows up influences their attitudes, values, customs, traditions and the language and dialect they speak. All these factors affect the way that an individual thinks, speaks and behaves. Should they move to a different area or another country, they will find that there will be differences between them and the local inhabitants.

Social class

Social class is the classification (grouping) of people according to their status in society. One way of grouping them is based on their occupations (jobs). Generally, occupations are linked to income, and people with a high income are likely to have more choices and a higher standard of living than those with lower incomes. Generally, those on low incomes are likely to have more ill-health and a shorter life span. National statistics about the social classes are useful for the government when making policy decisions to reduce the inequalities in society. (➲ page 68.)

Political factors

Political factors are those relating to government policies and legislation. **Legislation** is the making of laws and regulations by parliament including those that set out policy frameworks for the Welfare State.

The Welfare State

The Welfare State was set up by the government in 1948 to ensure a minimum standard of living for everyone. Money from taxation is used to provide welfare services:

- Social Security – financial help in the form of unemployment and sickness benefits, family allowances and income support;
- Social Services for people's general welfare (➲ p. 194);
- the National Health Service (NHS ➲ p. 199);
- education;
- social housing;
- public libraries;
- subsidised public transport and leisure facilities with special discounts for the elderly, unemployed and disabled.

3. a In what ways may a person be influenced by the place where they grew up?

b What is meant by social class?

c Describe the link between:
  i high income and health,
  ii low income and health.

d When can statistics about social class be useful?

e What are political factors?

f i Why was the Welfare State set up,
  ii where did the money come from,
  iii what welfare services were provided?

Equality

Whatever their personal differences, people are entitled to equality of treatment by the health and social care services. Care workers are expected to be **non-discriminatory**, which means treating everyone equally whatever their age, gender, race, disability, culture, religion or class.

Discrimination

Discrimination occurs when one person is treated less fairly than another. The unfair treatment can be based on prejudice, stereotyping or labelling.

Prejudice means having biased opinions that favour or disfavour individuals or groups of people. Prejudice is not based on personal experience or good evidence, but on other people's opinions or those of the media.

Stereotyping is putting people into groups based on one or more features that they are assumed to have in common.

Labelling is a one-word or brief description applied to a person. It identifies that person as being of a certain type whether it is true or untrue. Labels that are wrongly used can be very hurtful to the person concerned, and often intended to be so.

Laws to promote equality

To prevent discrimination, parliament has passed a number of laws that apply to everyone. These laws apply to both the people employed in the health and social care services and to service users. They enable individuals to lodge complaints when they experience discrimination on the grounds of:

- unequal pay for men and women (Equal Pay Act 1970);
- sex, gender or marital status (Sex Discrimination Act 1975);
- race, colour or nationality (Race Relations Act 2000);
- disability (Disability Discrimination Act 1995);
- sexual orientation, religion or belief, or age (Employment Equality Regulations);
- loss of rights and freedoms (Human Rights Act 1998);

Laws to promote equality are discussed further on pages 84-85.

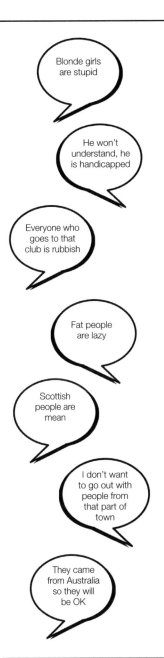

Blonde girls are stupid

He won't understand, he is handicapped

Everyone who goes to that club is rubbish

Fat people are lazy

Scottish people are mean

I don't want to go out with people from that part of town

They came from Australia so they will be OK

---

4. a What is meant by:
  i discrimination;
  ii non-discrimination.
  b Explain the difference between:
  i prejudice; **ii** stereotyping;
  iii labelling. Add an example.
  c Which of the laws to prevent discrimination might apply when a person was told that they were unsuitable to be employed because:
  i they were too old;
  ii they were married;
  iii they were homosexual;
  iv they had a disability;
  v of their religion?

Activities

1. Using the media, find examples of unfair treatment of people because of their age, disability, gender, sexual orientation, race or nationality, religion or belief or loss of rights. (➲ Media search page 245)
2. Interview a care worker to find out how unfair treatment can be prevented in health and social care organisations.

Care Value Base

Care values

Care values are beliefs about the correct way for care workers to treat people receiving care – the service users (patients and clients). The care values form the **Care Value Base** which is a set of values and principles for health and social care workers.

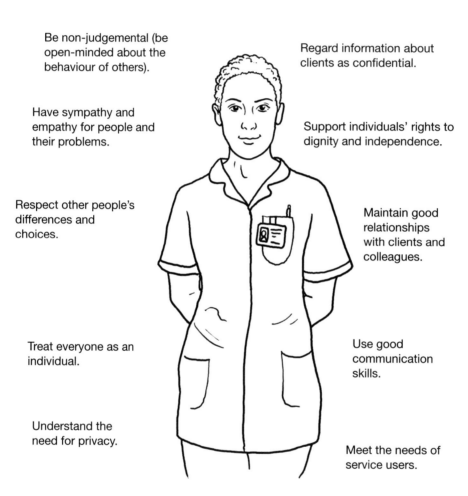

Be non-judgemental (be open-minded about the behaviour of others).

Have sympathy and empathy for people and their problems.

Respect other people's differences and choices.

Treat everyone as an individual.

Understand the need for privacy.

Regard information about clients as confidential.

Support individuals' rights to dignity and independence.

Maintain good relationships with clients and colleagues.

Use good communication skills.

Meet the needs of service users.

Care Value Base

Activity

Ten care values are shown above. From your own experience, record an occasion when each care value applied. It could be your behaviour towards someone else or their behaviour towards you. For example, it could be an occasion when you needed privacy or when you had sympathy for someone else's problems.

1. a i What are care values?
   ii List ten care values.
   b i What is the Care Value Base,
   ii who is it intended for?

Codes of practice

A **code of practice** contains guidelines for how people should carry out their duties and how they should behave. Different sectors of the caring services have their own codes of practice, for example the:

- **Nursing and Midwifery Council (NMC)** for nurses and midwives;
- **General Social Care Council (GSCC)** for social care. The GSCC has produced two codes of practice, one for social care workers and the other for the employers of social care workers. Both are described below.

CODE OF PRACTICE FOR EMPLOYERS OF SOCIAL CARE WORKERS

Social care employers must:

- make sure that people are suitable to enter the workforce and able to understand their roles and responsibilities.
- have written policies and procedures in place to enable social care workers to meet the GSCC's Code of Practice for Social Care Workers (➲ see the column on the right);
- provide training and development opportunities to enable social care workers to strengthen and develop their skills and knowledge;
- put into place and implement written policies and procedures to deal with dangerous, discriminatory or exploitative behaviour and practice;
- promote the GSCC's codes of practice to social care workers, service users and carers and cooperate with the GSCC's proceedings.

CODE OF PRACTICE FOR SOCIAL CARE WORKERS

Social care workers must:

- protect the rights and promote the interests of service users and carers;
- strive to establish and maintain the trust and confidence of service users and carers;
- promote the independence of service users while protecting them as far as possible from danger and harm;
- respect the rights of service users while seeking to ensure that their behaviour does not harm themselves or other people;
- uphold public trust and confidence in social care services;
- be accountable for the quality of their work and take responsibility for maintaining and improving their knowledge and skills.

Activity

a Make a list of what you think are the key points in the Nursing Code of Practice.
b Which of your points are similar to those points included in the Code of Practice for Social Workers?
c Which of your points are different from those points included in the Code of Practice for Social Workers?
d What conclusions do you draw from comparing these two documents?

2. a What is the purpose of a code of practice?
   b Name a code of practice that applies in the NHS.
   c What does GSCC stand for?
   d Before social care workers are employed, what must employers ensure?
   e What written policies must employers have for their social care workers?
   f To develop skills and knowledge, what is required of:
      i employers of social care workers;
      ii social care workers themselves?

Vulnerable service users

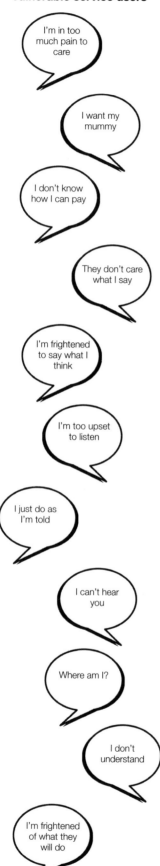

Policies and charters

The Department of Health is responsible for the policies in health and social care in England and Wales. These policies set standards in all areas of the NHS, in social care and in public health. Individual organisations may produce charters to inform service users of their rights and the service they can expect to receive from that organisation.

Care workers' responsibilities

Care workers are responsible for providing a service that upholds the individual rights of service users, which involves giving them **active support** by:

- listening to their needs, views and preferences;
- overcoming communication barriers;
- being non-judgemental;
- providing practical care when needed;
- understanding the needs and feelings of vulnerable people.

Vulnerable service users

People who need care are often **vulnerable** – easily hurt and with poor defences, for example:

- poor eyesight or hearing;
- feeling inferior to people in authority;
- a feeling of being unable to change things;
- they cannot understand what is said to them;
- too nervous to express their thoughts and feelings;
- too distressed to understand what is being said to them;
- too ill to cooperate;
- confused by unfamiliar surroundings;
- afraid of what might happen to them;
- worried about money;
- too young to protest against unsuitable treatment.

Activities

1. Identify the principles of:
   i   the Care Value Base,
   ii care workers' responsibilities.
2. Give a talk of at least four minutes on 'Care workers' responsibilities'.
(➲ Giving a talk page 242.)

3. a i Who sets health and care policies in England,
   ii what is the purpose of these policies?
   b What is the purpose of charters?
   c How do carers provide active support for patients and clients?
   d What does being vulnerable mean? Give some examples.
   e In two columns, list the conditions that can make people vulnerable, then choose a speech bubble that illustrates it.

Individual rights

Charters and codes of practice for health and care services contain a range of rights that service users can expect to receive.

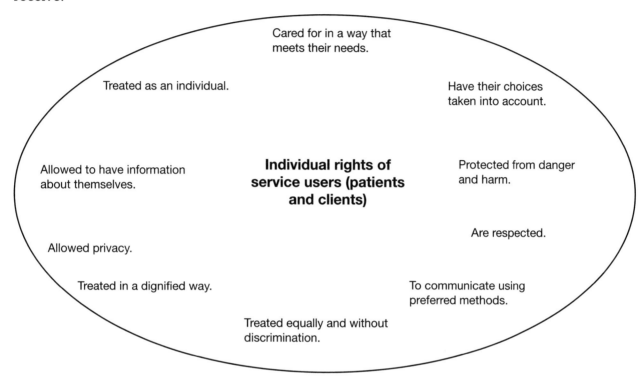

Cared for in a way that meets their needs.

Treated as an individual.

Have their choices taken into account.

Allowed to have information about themselves.

Individual rights of service users (patients and clients)

Protected from danger and harm.

Are respected.

Allowed privacy.

Treated in a dignified way.

To communicate using preferred methods.

Treated equally and without discrimination.

Individual responsibilities

Although people have their individual rights, they are also responsible for respecting the rights of other people. Rights and responsibilities therefore have to be balanced, and tensions occur when people see their rights and responsibilities differently. When differences do occur in a health and social care setting, service users act responsibly when they:

- keep calm as they explain their point;
- listen to another person's point of view;
- are prepared to accept the facts.

Examples of tensions between rights and responsibilities

Cause of tension	Rights	Responsibilities
Lack of privacy	to privacy	not to deny privacy to others
Antisocial behaviour	to be respected	to respect other people
Television on or off?	to watch television	not to disturb other people's peace

Activity

Describe the rights of patients/service users.

4. a i When people have rights, what responsibility do they also have,
ii when may tensions occur,
iii how can service users act responsibly?
b Compare the individual rights of service users with the care values expected of social care workers on page 18. Select five pairs of statements that have similar meanings (one from each group). List them in two columns:

Social workers' care values	Service users' rights

Confidentiality

Confidentiality means keeping information secret unless there is a very good reason for telling someone else. In order to do their job, care workers need to know a great deal of personal information about service users. It is essential that this is kept confidential by care workers because:

- it is a legal requirement to maintain the confidentiality of personal records;
- it encourages clients to trust care workers with personal Information;
- clients who know that their personal details will not become gossip are more likely to tell care workers what they really think and feel;
- a client's self esteem could be damaged by knowing that his/her personal details were public knowledge;
- confidential information passed to the wrong people might result in the client being treated unfairly.

Disclosure

Disclosure means revealing information to another person. Care workers should always ask service users for permission before passing on personal information about them. For example 'Do you mind if I tell your family that . . .'. They should also not let other people see personal records of patients or clients, nor talk about service user's private matters when others can overhear.

Disclosing confidential information

Although care workers are expected to regard information about service users as confidential, there will be times when it is necessary to inform their colleagues, managers or other professionals on a 'need to know basis'. This can occur when:

- clients are in danger of harming themselves or others;
- clients have broken, or are going to break, the law;
- managers need to be informed;
- other professionals need to be informed about a service user on a 'need to know' basis. Those who receive information on a 'need to know' basis will be expected to keep that information confidential.

Activity

Using a computer, design a poster on confidentiality for staff in a hospital. Include examples for each of the reasons for keeping information confidential given above.

5. **a** Explain the difference between confidentiality and disclosure.
   b Why is confidentiality essential in care work?
   c Name two actions that care workers can take to maintain confidentiality.
   d When may confidential information need to be disclosed?
   e How should 'need to know' information be treated?

Recording and retrieving information

Records are the way in which information is kept and they provide a historical account of what has occurred. They can be hand-written notes, electronic records or computer print-outs. They may be forms which have been filled in, records of meetings or events, medicines prescribed and treatment given, decisions made and information sent to service users. Records are legal documents and can be used in court cases if required.

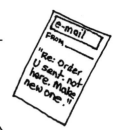

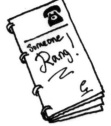

Keeping records

- **Accuracy** It is essential for records to be **accurate** – inaccurate information is useless, causes other people to waste time putting mistakes right, and can be dangerous if inaccurate information results in harm.
- **Correct filing** of paper records is essential so that they can be retrieved easily. When records are lost a large amount of time is spent looking for them.

Records should:

- contain the **date** of each entry, and sometimes also the **time**;
- be **signed** with a signature plus the printed name of the person responsible for the record with their job description;
- have any **alterations or updating** initialled and dated by the person who makes the changes.

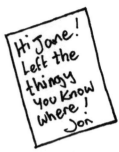

They should also:

- **be legible** – easy for other people to read;
- **be relevant** – include vital information and opinions but not unnecessary details;
- **not contain personal comments** or opinions;
- **be stored safely** – either manually in a filing system, or electronically in a computer or separate memory device.

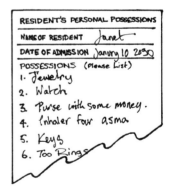

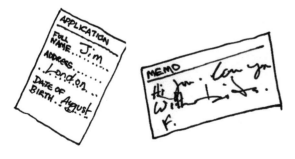

Activity

How many mistakes can you spot in the drawings of records on this page?

6. **a** What are records?
   b What different forms can records take?
   c Why do records need to be accurate?
   d Why do paper records need to be filed correctly?
   e Because records can be used as legal documents:
      i what must they contain,
      ii how should they be signed,
      iii what must happen if they are altered?
   f When are records
      i legible,
      ii relevant.
   g How should records be stored?

NHS Care Records Service

The NHS is working towards an electronic system that stores all patients' records digitally. It will contain a complete medical history of each patient including health problems, test results, scans, X-rays, dates of vaccinations, diagnoses, letters to the patient, medicines prescribed, drug reactions, and any in-patient or out-patient hospital care. The service is intended to:

- reduce form-filling for patients and NHS staff;
- provide basic information that will not have to be repeatedly given to different members of the NHS staff;
- give NHS staff 24-hour access to up-to-date, accurate information about the patient, hopefully making diagnosis and treatment safer and faster;
- maintain confidentiality by only allowing access to patients' records on a strictly 'need to know' basis.

The Data Protection Act

The Data Protection Act 1998 is an act of parliament that gives people the right to access information held about themselves by organisations. Clients can access personal information held by social service and housing departments. Patients are able to access their medical reports for a small fee.

Activities

1. Complete a table that lists service users' rights and the corresponding care workers' responsibilities.
2. Use examples to explain how the Care Value Base and care workers' responsibilities promote service users' rights.

7. **a** What will an electronic patient record contain?
   b What are the benefits of an electronic patient record system?
   c What is the purpose of the Data Protection Act?

Chapter 2
Individual Needs

This chapter covers:

- The everyday needs of individuals in society.

- Factors that influence the health and needs of individuals.

- Hazards in health and social care environments.

- Health and safety legislation and guidelines.

The needs of individuals in society

Maslow's hierarchy

Abraham Maslow is famous for his theory of 'The hierarchy of human needs' published in 1943. It was based on the knowledge that everyone has needs - for survival, protection from harm, friendship, self-esteem and the need to belong and to achieve. He placed these in a pyramid with the most basic human needs necessary for survival at the bottom. He reasoned that the needs lower down in the pyramid were the most important and had to be satisfied before those higher up could be realised. The highest need is the personal fulfilment (self-actualisation) that comes from making the most of your abilities and skills.

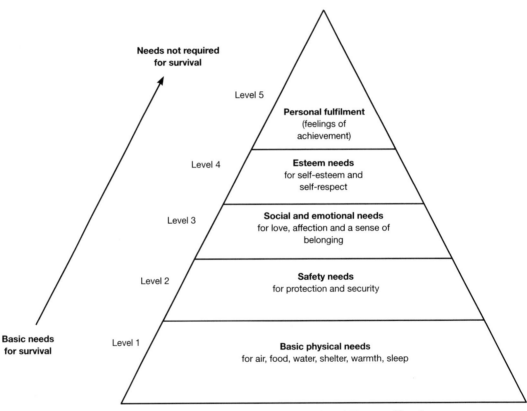

Maslow's Hierarchy of Human Needs

Activity

What are your personal needs? List them then put them into the five groups above.

1. **a** What is Maslow's theory based on?
   b Draw a diagram of Maslow's hierarchy of human needs.
   c Why did Maslow place physical needs at the bottom of the pyramid?

Physical and safety needs

Physical needs are those concerned with staying alive:

- **water** for drinking and keeping clean;
- **food** for growth, energy and health;
- **shelter** from the weather;
- **warmth** to help keep the body at a suitable temperature;
- **sleep** to restore the body and mind.

An individual who is hungry, thirsty and cold will have an over-riding desire to find food, water, shelter and warmth in order to survive. When these basic needs have been met, **personal safety** then becomes important. When safe from danger and harm, people can feel secure. Long-term feelings of insecurity can damage a person's physical and mental health.

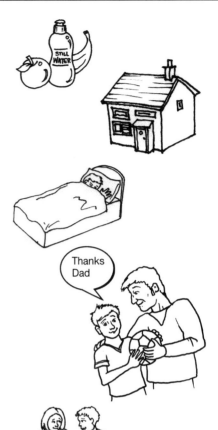

Social needs

Social needs are met by contact with other people. For example:

- being part of a family group;
- enjoying the company of colleagues at work;
- belonging to groups, clubs and religious organisations;
- mixing with others at meetings, parties, outings, cafes, bars and restaurants;
- having friends and good relationships with others.

Relationships

Relationships are personal links with other people. **A good relationship** depends on trust. It results in healthy, positive feelings of confidence, willingness to share, pleasure in the company of people who can be depended on for support and a sense of belonging and acceptance.

A poor relationship is one in which people do not trust each other. Confidence is lost, there is no willingness to share things, and no enjoyment in the company of people who cannot be trusted. It results in negative feelings of anger and resentment.

Working relationships develop among people who work together. People in a **good working relationship** feel valued and get more enjoyment out of their jobs and with less stress. In a **poor working relationship** people feel unvalued and unhappy, and there is an increase in absence from work due to stress-related illness or malingering (pretending to be ill).

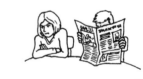

2. **a** List five physical needs and explain why each is necessary.
   b **i** When do people feel secure,
      ii why can insecurity be harmful?
   c How are social needs met?
   d What is a relationship?
   e Compare a good relationship with a poor relationship.
   f Compare the effects of a good working relationship with a poor working relationship.
   g Which needs are illustrated on this page?
   h What types of relationship are illustrated on this page?

> ## Activity
>
> Describe how you feel when you are: **i** cold and hungry; **ii** in a good relationship with someone; **iii** rejected by someone you considered a friend; **iv** being praised for an achievement; **v** lonely.

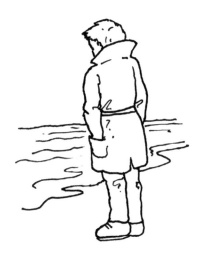

Emotional needs

Emotions are feelings. People's emotional needs are met by **positive emotions** that come from love and affection, friendships and relationships that are secure. Positive emotions make people feel wanted, valued and contented.

Negative emotions include fear, anger, anxiety, depression, boredom, loneliness, insecurity and low self-esteem. When negative emotions dominate a person's life they can give rise to smouldering resentment or outbursts of aggression, and put a great strain on relationships.

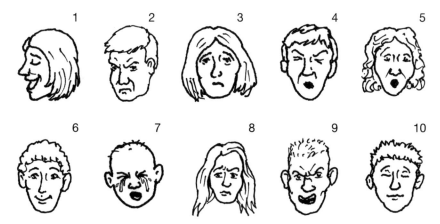

Loneliness

Loneliness (social isolation) is being cut-off from enough contact with other people. Although a few people prefer their own company and enjoy being alone, most suffer from loneliness when too much time is spent on their own. Lonely people can become very depressed and lose interest in what they do or eat, and their health may suffer. For example, this can happen when a teenager is bullied and isolated and has no-one to turn to for support; or in old age, when it becomes physically and mentally difficult to contact people.

Activities

1. **a** Sort the ten faces above into emotions that show:
   amusement   distress
   happiness   rage   anger
   pain   fear   sadness
   doubt   contentment
   b For each give an occasion when your face could show a similar emotion.
2. Mrs X lives on her own in a small town. She says she doesn't like or need people, doesn't want anything to do with them, and prefers the company of her cats. Can Mrs X live without other people? Explain your answer.
3. Discuss situations in life than can result in loneliness, ways of overcoming loneliness, and the organisations that offer support to lonely people.
   (➲ page 243 'Discussion'.)

3. **a** What are emotions?
   i Give examples of positive emotions,
   ii Give examples of negative emotions,
   iii Compare the effects of positive and negative feelings.
   b What is loneliness,
   i how can it affect people,
   ii why is it more common in old age?

Intellectual needs

The thinking part of the **brain** (the intellect) needs the stimulation of activities that are interesting or new. Children meet their intellectual needs by learning through play, asking questions and exploring their environment. Older children and adults fulfil their intellectual needs in many ways. It may be by having a particular interest or hobby, the challenge of passing exams, winning a game, completing a task, or the esteem that comes from doing a job they enjoy and for which they are valued. When the mind is not regularly stimulated it becomes sluggish and reluctant to work. The brain can also be damaged by too much alcohol and by other drug use.

Boredom

People become bored when their intellectual needs are not met. **Boredom** is a state of being tired and uninterested in anything due to being mentally under-occupied. Some young people escape from boredom by developing restless, challenging behaviour or by becoming involved in gang culture. For people of any age, long-term boredom can become a health risk when it results in low self-esteem and depression, or in activities to relieve the boredom such as just sitting all day in front of a TV set, over-eating, smoking, alcohol or drug abuse.

Activity

Joe is 16 and homeless. He lives on the streets in a city far from his home town. He ran away from his violent father. You find Joe in a doorway on the coldest night of the year.

Mary has dementia and has just been moved into a care home after her husband died. Her only daughter and her family moved to Australia two years ago. Mary seems distressed and unhappy.

Amir has recently arrived in England from Iraq. He has found a place to live but he doesn't know anyone in the local area. He doesn't speak English and he is working in a factory making clothes. In Iraq he had trained to be a doctor.

1. Make a list of the every-day physical needs of Joe, Mary and Amir.
2. Considering Joe, Mary and Amir separately:
   a Which social needs are not being met?
   b Which emotional needs are not being met?
   c Which intellectual needs are not being met?
3. What would you suggest doing to meet the needs of Joe, Mary and Amir?
4. Which organisations would you suggest contacting for advice?
5. Identify four factors that may have influenced the health and needs of Joe, Mary and Amir.

4. a What stimulates the brain?
   b How are intellectual needs met by:
      i children,
      ii adults?
   c i When do people become bored?
      ii Describe the state of boredom.
      iii How may some young people react to boredom?
      iv What are the dangers of long-term boredom?

Factors that influence the health and needs of the individuals

The **World Health Organisation** (WHO) defines **health** as 'a state of complete physical, mental and social well-being and not merely the absence of disease and infirmity'. **Well-being** is a feeling of control over your life and optimism about the future.

Factors that have an influence on health and well-being can be classed as physical (➲ below), socio-economic (➲ page 31), lifestyle (➲ page 36) and abuse (➲ page 47).

Physical factors

Physical factors are those relating to the body rather than the mind. They are the result of the interaction of inherited and environmental factors.

Inherited factors (genes)

Inherited factors are the genes inherited from parents. Each child inherits one set of genes from the mother and another set from the father. Together they provide instructions for growth and development of a new individual. For example, they determine the gender (male or female), hair colour, eye colour, blood group, foot size, shape of nose, the maximum height that a child can grow, and whether it is possible to 'roll the tongue'.

Inherited diseases are due to defective genes that are passed from parents to children. Examples are cystic fibrosis, muscular dystrophy, haemophilia and some forms of breast cancer.

Environmental factors

Environment means the surrounding conditions. Environmental conditions that affect health and well-being include:

- **air quality** Air polluted by traffic fumes and smoke from cigarettes and factory chimneys can cause respiratory diseases and cancer.
- **water supplies** Water is essential for life. Tap water is treated to make it safe for drinking and to prevent water-borne diseases such as E.coli, typhoid and cholera. Water is also needed to keep the environment clean and for industry and farming.
- housing (➲ page 32).

1. a What does WHO stand for, and how does it define health?
   b What does 'well-being' mean?
   c What are physical factors?
   d i Where do a person's genes come from,
     ii what is their function?
   e i What causes inherited diseases?
     ii Give three examples.
   f What is the environment?
   g Give reasons why air quality is important.
   h i Give three uses for water.
     ii Why is tap water treated?

Socio-economic factors

Socio-economic factors are those that refer to the social and economic aspects of people's lives and include social class, employment, housing, income, education, access to services, media, gender, culture and religion.

Social class

Social class is a way of placing people into groups who share a similar position in society. It is linked with income, occupation and lifestyle. Generally, people in a higher social class have more money, power, influence and better health than those in the lower classes. (➲ page 68.)

Employment

Employment can mean paid work or voluntary work – volunteering to do a job without pay. Being employed is usually healthier for people than being unemployed.

Unemployment is linked to poor physical and mental health. Those in work tend to live longer than those without jobs. Unemployed men and women are more likely to die from heart disease, accidents and suicide than those in work.

Work-related stress occurs when a worker is under too much pressure for one reason or another. People work best when they are under a moderate amount of pressure. Too little pressure results in boredom; too much can contribute to health problems. (➲ page 40.)

Social exclusion

Social exclusion means being unable to access the things in life that most people take for granted. This may happen to alcoholics and drug addicts who are poor and unemployed, homeless and without family or friends. They might not be registered with a GP (doctor), and may not have access to the health and social services they need. All these factors make it difficult for them to form normal relationships with other people, and they become isolated in society.

2. a Name ten socio-economic factors.
   b i What is social class,
     ii what is it linked to?
   c How may the classes differ?
   d Name two types of employment.
   e What is unemployment linked with?
   f Explain why work is said to be good for health?
   g i When do people work best,
     ii what is work-related stress?
     iii what results from too little stress?
   h Describe the effects of social exclusion.

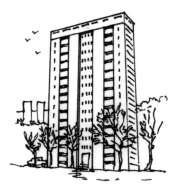

High-rise tower blocks can lead to social isolation when:
- the neighbours are rarely seen;
- when the lifts do not work;
- when people are fearful of leaving their homes;
- children cannot play safely outside.

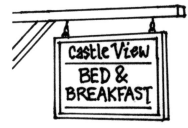

Bed and breakfast hotels provide only temporary accommodation and are unsuitable for families.

Activities

1. Research homelessness in your area to give a talk on the subject for at least four minutes. For example, how many people are homeless? Where can they go for advice? Are there any local organisations that help homeless people? (➲ page 242 'Giving a talk'.)

2. **Shelter** is a national charity for housing and homelessness. From its website, find out who founded it, its vision and what it does.

Housing and health

The type of housing that people live in is usually related to their income. Families on low incomes are less likely to own their own homes or have the money to keep them in good condition. They are more likely to live in damp, overcrowded and neglected property that can be a cause of ill-health to people of all ages. For example:

- **cold and damp conditions** can aggravate illnesses such as arthritis, rheumatism and asthma, bronchitis and pneumonia.
- **overcrowding** can result in sleeplessness, stress and depression, encourage the spread of infectious diseases and make accidents more likely.
- **childrens' education** is adversely affected as overcrowded conditions means fewer opportunities to play or study.

Homelessness

In 2006, it was estimated that the UK had more than 400,000 homeless people from many different backgrounds and ethnic groups. Homelessness is rarely a lifestyle choice. It is often the result of unemployment and financial hardship, relationship breakdown, domestic violence, health problems, mental illness and substance abuse, usually alcohol.

People who are homeless may be able to stay with family or friends, the local authority (council) may be able to re-house them or provide bed-and-breakfast accommodation, or they may find a place in a hostel. When these possibilities fail, often due to misbehaviour, the only option left is to sleep rough.

Sleeping rough on park benches, street doorways or wherever a space can be found, makes homeless people prone to poor physical and mental health. Because they do not have an address they have difficulty in getting jobs and face difficulties in getting the financial and emotional support that they need.

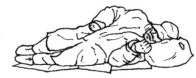

Sleeping rough is the last resort for those without money or support from family or friends.

3. a i In what way is housing related to income,
     ii how can cold, damp conditions affect health,
     iii what are the effects of over-crowding?
   b How may a child's education be affected by bad housing?
   c Why do people become homeless?
   d What are the options for homeless people?
   e What difficulties are faced by people who sleep rough?
   f In what ways may tower blocks lead to social isolation?

Income

Income is the money received by a person or a family over a period of time from:

- working;
- pensions such as retirement pensions;
- savings and investments;
- welfare benefits such as child benefit, unemployment benefit, housing benefit and disablement benefits.

Money is needed to pay for essentials such as food, clothing, housing and warmth. People in **absolute poverty** do not have enough money to pay for these essential items. This is rare in the UK because there are welfare benefits for those with little or no income. **Relative poverty** is more common. It means not having the goods, services and pleasures that other people take for granted. Those most likely to be in this group are:

- pensioners;
- people with disabilities;
- lone parent families;
- families where the breadwinner is unemployed.

Income and health

There is a strong link between poverty and health. More people on low incomes have health problems than those who are better off.

- **Physical ill-health** can be caused by poor housing conditions, poor diet and lack of enough heat to keep warm.
- **Mental ill-health** can be due to the stress of 'trying to make ends meet' for years on end. It is difficult to take part in activities enjoyed by most other people, and there is never enough money for luxuries, holidays or outings. The result can be feelings of isolation, unhappiness, boredom and depression.
- **Life expectancy** There are big differences in life expectancy and disease rates between people living in wealthy areas and those living in the poor areas.

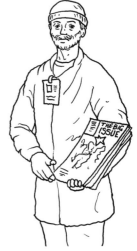

The *Big Issue* magazine is a news and current affairs magazine written by professional journalists. It is sold on the streets by people who are homeless. This gives them the opportunity to earn an income and regain self-esteem and the dignity of independence.

4. **a** Name four possible sources of income.
   b **i** Describe the difference between absolute poverty and relative poverty.
   ii Which groups of people are more likely to be relatively poor?
   c How may a low income affect:
   i physical health,
   ii mental health,
   iii life expectancy?
   d **i** What is the *Big Issue*
   ii who sells it,
   iii who benefits?

Activities

1. Find out:
   a Which welfare benefits are available from social security for people who are unemployed?
   b Where does the money come from to pay for welfare benefits?
2. Poverty is to do with money, not values. A person who is poor may be of great value to their family, friends and society. Discuss: 'Is it better to be poor and happy or rich and unhappy?' (➔ page 243 'Discussion'.)

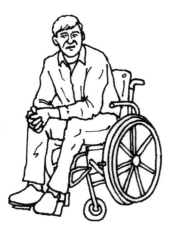

Tom came from a low-income family, never went to nursery or playschool, didn't like school, often played truant and became used to long-term unemployment. He drinks and smokes to relieve the boredom and, since his stroke, has been confined to a wheelchair.

5. **a** What is the purpose of educating children?
   b In what way could Tom have benefited from pre-school education?
   c What are the benefits that Tom could have received from a good education?
   d What is low-achievement at school closely linked with?
   e Describe five barriers that could prevent Tom from accessing the care services he needs after he had his stroke.
   f What is the media and what does it do?
   g In what ways may health topics be reported?

Activity

Collect some news items and stories about health topics from different sources. Select three and, for each, give your opinion on the way it was reported by comparing it with the five possible influences of the media listed above.

Education

An appropriate education prepares children for the world of work so that they can provide for themselves and their families. It also gives them the information and confidence to make healthy lifestyle choices. Low achievement at school is closely linked with truancy, teenage pregnancy, unemployment, higher rates of disease and shorter life expectancy.

Children, especially those from disadvantaged backgrounds, who experience good pre-school education are better prepared for school and learn more quickly.

Access to services

Barriers that can prevent patients from accessing the services they need are:

- **physical barriers** – steps and stairs too difficult to climb and doorways too narrow for wheelchairs;
- **location** – when there is no transport, or it is too far to travel;
- **financial barriers** – patients cannot afford to pay for the service or the travel costs;
- **the required service is not available in the district** although it is available for people living in other districts – this is known as the **postcode lottery**;
- **lack of knowledge** – people do not know the service exists;
- **culture** – people who are too shy or fearful of strangers or unfamiliar places, or who find it difficult to make themselves understood, or are prevented by their religion.

Media

The **mass media** includes television, radio, newspapers, magazines and mass advertisements. It communicates information to a mass audience (the general public) and is influential in shaping public opinion. For example, depending on how health topics are reported, they can:

- **make people aware of health issues** such as testicular cancer;
- **create health scares**, making people worry about their health;
- **raise false hopes** about health 'cures' before the research has been completed and the treatment tested;
- **reduce prejudice** surrounding mental health and disabilities;
- **increase prejudice** against mental illness and disabilities.

Gender

Whether a baby is born a boy or a girl depends on their genes. Their **gender** (**sex**) is either male or female, but their gender identity may be different. **Gender identity** is the gender to which a person feels he or she belongs. For example, a biological male may wish to live as a woman or a biological female may wish to live as a man.

Gender roles are the attitudes and behaviours that are considered more appropriate for one gender or the other within a culture. They vary from one culture to another, and from one religion to another.

In general, males:
- are expected to be brave and not cry;
- take more interest in sports;
- are more aggressive and play fighting games;
- earn more;
- are more interested in machinery and the way things work;
- are convicted more often of crimes, especially crimes involving violence and/or sex.

In general, females:
- are expected to be more emotional;
- take more responsibility for child-rearing;
- do most of the household chores;
- achieve better grades at school;
- earn less;
- have greater life-expectancy.

Culture

The **culture** (customs) of any particular social group can affect the health and needs of its members. For example:

- the custom of sunbathing can result in skin cancer;
- the custom of covering the skin from sunlight can result in rickets in children and softening of the bones (**osteomalacia**) in adults;
- the fast food culture is linked with obesity;
- a culture that admires very thin women many encourage anorexia.

Religion

Each religion has its own set of beliefs and views on behaviour. These can include diet, dress, gender roles and type of worship. People from different cultural backgrounds may have quite different attitudes and behaviour from those working in health and care settings. Awareness of the importance of personal beliefs and the religions of patients and clients is a key requirement for care workers. (➲ pages 78-82.)

6. **a** What is meant by:
   i gender,
   ii gender identity,
   iii gender roles?
b Name some gender characteristics for:
   i males,
   ii females.
c Give examples of links between culture and health.
d i What may distinguish one religion from another.
   ii what is a key requirement for care workers?

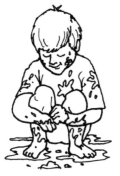

Building up immunity
Young children need to be kept clean, but not too clean. Contact with small doses of germs enables them to build up immunity against infectious diseases.

Activity

Find information about MRSA and C. difficile. Then make notes on each infection to describe:
i   how the infection spreads;
ii the actions taken to reduce infection.

Lifestyle factors

Lifestyle is the way in which a person chooses to live their life. Lifestyle factors include personal hygiene, diet, exercise, posture, stress, substance abuse, alcohol, smoking and sexual health. People's lifestyles and the conditions in which they work strongly influence their health.

Hygiene

Hygiene is concerned with cleanliness to prevent the spread of infectious diseases. Infectious diseases are caused by **germs** (microbes) especially bacteria or viruses. Germs can spread rapidly in places such as hospitals and residential homes due to:

- warm conditions that encourage the spread of infectious diseases brought in by patients or visitors;
- the close contact of patients or residents and their carers.

Clean environmental conditions are particularly important for:

- **babies** as they are still developing immunity;
- **sick people** whose immunity has been lowered by illness;
- **older people** as they often have reduced immunity.

Personal hygiene is essential for people who work closely with other people as germs can spread quickly from one person to another. This applies to health and social care workers as many of their patients or clients are vulnerable to infection unless strict hygiene rules are followed.

Clean clothing.

Wash hands after using the toilet.

Keep nails short and clean and don't wear false nails.

Wash regularly to remove sweat and dirt.

Personal hygiene for health and care workers

Use a paper handkerchief when sneezing and coughing and dispose of it safely.

Clean teeth properly.

Use a deodorant.

Cover cuts with a clean dressing.

Clean, tidy hair, and long hair tied back.

Wash hands thoroughly between tasks, or use disinfectant gel.

---

7. **a** What is the purpose of hygiene?
   b Which groups of people need clean environmental conditions and why?
   c Why is too much cleanliness not good for young children?
   d Why is good personal hygiene important for health and care workers?
   e List the requirements of personal hygiene for health and care workers.

Poor personal hygiene

People who do not wash themselves or their clothes often enough give off a smell that most other people find unpleasant. Smelly people are therefore avoided and become socially isolated. The smells from unwashed people come from bacteria living on the skin and in clothes. The bacteria survive on:

- moisture from sweat;
- food from the skin surface, sweat, urine and dirt;
- warmth from body heat.

Washing removes dirt from the skin together with most of the bacteria that naturally live there. Some bacteria are essential to keep the skin healthy, and it is impossible to wash them all off, or even scrub them off.

Body odour The warm, moist conditions of the armpits, bottom and feet are ideal for bacteria and they quickly grow and multiply. In doing so, smells are produced known as body odour. Body odour can be prevented from building up to an unpleasant level by regularly washing the body, particularly the more smelly areas, and the clothes worn next to the skin.

Bad breath (halitosis)

Temporary causes include uncleaned teeth, smoking, the recent eating of garlic, onions or other strongly flavoured food.

Persistent causes include rotting teeth and gum infections, sinusitis, bronchitis, indigestion and constipation.

Human parasites

Humans provide a source of food for a number of parasites. In the right conditions, they spread easily from one person to another, but do not survive long on clean people or in clean homes.

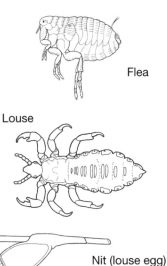

Flea

Louse

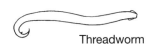

Nit (louse egg)

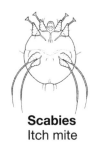

Threadworm

Scabies
Itch mite

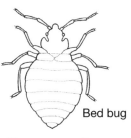

Bed bug

Human parasites
(Not to scale)

8. **a** What are the effects of poor personal hygiene?
   b Where do the smells from unwashed people come from?
   c From where do skin bacteria obtain water, food and warmth?
   d How does washing affect skin bacteria?
   e i How is body odour produced,
     ii how can it be controlled?
   f i How can care workers prevent temporary bad breath,
     ii What are the causes of permanent bad breath?
   g Why do parasites live on humans?

Activity

For each of the five parasites shown here, find out:
- where they live,
- what they feed on,
- where they lay their eggs,
- how they pass from one person to another,
- how they can be eradicated.

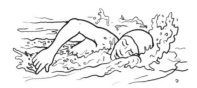

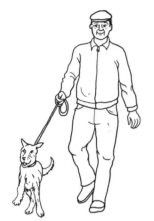

Swimming exercises most of the body's muscles.

Walking briskly for half an hour, five times a week, reduces the risk of heart disease.

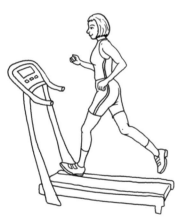

Aerobic exercise for at least 20 minutes, two or three times a week, improves stamina and endurance.

Exercise

People who exercise regularly usually feel fitter and have fewer days off sick than those who do not. This is because exercise:

- uses muscles and keeps them in good condition;
- keep joints flexible and improves posture;
- increases the rate and depth of breathing and oxygen intake;
- improves circulation and helps to keep the heart healthy;
- helps to control body weight by burning up fat;
- improves quality of life in later years.

Effects on the brain

Exercise can help to relieve depression and provide natural pain relief by releasing:

- **serotonin** – a chemical that lifts the mood;
- **endorphins** – hormones that block pain signals in the brain.

Types of exercise

The amount and type of exercise suitable for each individual depends on age, physical fitness and state of training.

Gentle exercise such as walking maintains muscle strength and joint mobility and is suitable for everyone.

Moderate exercise raises the heart rate enough to improve circulation during a brisk walk, cycling slowly, leisurely swimming, dancing, table tennis or active gardening.

Aerobic exercise (cardiovascular exercise) results in deep, fast breathing and raises the heart rate. This causes blood to circulate quickly round the body and deliver more oxygen to the muscles when, for example, jogging, cycling, swimming, table tennis, football or an exercise class.

Strenuous exercise puts excessive pressure on muscles and joints and demands stamina and endurance. The risk of injury is much greater in those who are unfit.

9. **a** Give two usual effects of regular exercise.
   b Give the benefits of exercise on:
      i muscles; **ii** joints; **iii** breathing; **iv** circulation; **v** body weight;
      vi quality of life.
   c Describe two effects of exercise on the brain.
   d Name an exercise suitable for all.
   e Compare moderate exercise with aerobic exercise for their effects on circulation.
   f Describe a type of exercise that:
      i benefits the heart; **ii** improves stamina; **iii** involves most muscles.
   g **i** Give the effects of strenuous exercise; **ii** Who has the greater risk of injury?

Posture

Posture is the way the body is held when standing, sitting, walking, bending or lifting. **Good posture** allows the body to move easily and without putting undue strain on the muscles. **Poor posture** puts the muscles out of balance and gives rise to a wide range of common ailments such as back pain or stiff neck.

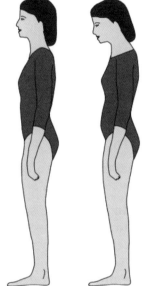

Head up.

Shoulders held back in a relaxed manner.

Backbone held in its correct shape.

Abdominal (tummy) muscles held in firmly.

Muscles of the thighs, legs and ankles are in balance.

Weight is well-balanced on the feet.

A drooping head tenses the neck muscles, causes a stiff neck and interferes with free movement of the head.

Rounded or hunched shoulders reduce space in the rib cage and restrict breathing.

A deep hollow in the back can cause pain in the back and/or legs.

Weak abdominal muscles give no support to the backbone.

Lop-sided standing puts extra strain on the muscles of the thighs, legs and ankles, making them ache.

Uneven distribution of weight on the feet makes them ache.

Good posture　　**Poor posture**

Back pain can develop gradually and get worse over months or years, for example when repeatedly using the wrong type of chair. It may also begin suddenly if the wrong posture is used when lifting or bending.

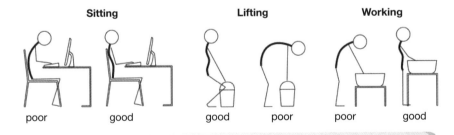

Sitting　　**Lifting**　　**Working**

poor　　good　　good　　poor　　poor　　good

10. a i What is meant by posture?
    ii What are the benefits of good posture?
    iii What are the effects of poor posture?
  b Create a table to compare good posture with poor posture for head, shoulders, backbone, abdominal muscles, legs, feet.
  c Under the heading 'Good posture', make three 'pinmen' drawings to illustrate sitting, lifting and working.
  d Under the heading 'Poor posture' make three 'pinmen' drawings to illustrate sitting, lifting and working.
  e Describe two ways in which back pain develops.

Activity

Comparing the good posture with poor posture, which in your opinion:
i is more attractive,
ii will give a better impression at interview,
iii is likely to make the job as a carer easier?
Give your reasons in each case.

Stressful events
Death of a relative, friend or pet.
Overwork.
Money worries.
Fear of having a serious illness.
Family disagreements.
Lack of sleep.
Moving house.
Seeing a serious accident.

Activity

A number of events that can be the cause of stress are named above. Use the internet to find organisations that can help people suffering from these causes of stress. Then give a talk for at least four minutes on your findings. (➲ page 242 'Giving a talk'.)

Stress

Moderate pressure helps to motivate people to achieve what they wish to do such as pass an exam, win a race or get a job. But too much pressure, or prolonged pressure, causes stress and affects health.

Effects of stress

Stress can cause symptoms such as:

- headache
- insomnia
- chest pains
- depression
- constant tiredness
- breathlessness
- abdominal pain
- lack of appetite
- nausea
- skin rash
- anxiety
- obesity

Stress can also make other disorders worse, for example asthma and migraine.

Strategies for coping with stress

Knowing what to do when becoming angry, upset or over-anxious helps to reduce a stressful situation. For example:

- **count up to ten** before saying or doing anything;
- **breathe slowly and deeply** until feeling calmer;
- **relax muscles** that have become tense, including face muscles;
- **take 'time out'** from the stressful situation for a short while;
- **identify the cause(s)** and take remedial action such as a healthier diet, a change of job or lifestyle, reducing the workload, taking more exercise or having a better social life and more fun.

Professional treatment

An important step in dealing with stress is for the person to admit that there is a problem and that professional help is needed. This can involve:

- **counselling** by people trained to deal with stress conditions to identify the cause(s) of the stress and advise on ways of dealing with it - in some cases, this is all the treatment that is needed;
- **group therapy** – meetings with people who have similar problems to discuss experiences;
- **medicines** such as anti-depressants for a limited time only.

11. a What can be the effect of:
    i moderate pressure, ii too much pressure?
   b Sort the symptoms of stress into 'physical' and 'mental'.
   c Name two disorders that can be made worse by stress.
   d Name three types of treatment for stress.
   e Describe some strategies for coping with stress.

Relaxation

Life in health and care settings is stressful at times for both carers and service users. Knowing how to relax in stressful situations enables people to think more clearly and to work more effectively.

Relaxation is time away from work or activity and it can be both physical and mental. Having a relaxed mind and body helps to calm anxious thoughts. It may not prevent the thoughts but it is a basis for getting some control over them.

- **Relaxation of the body** Move to a quiet place for a few minutes, make yourself comfortable, and breathe slowly and quietly. These all help to relax the muscles.
- **Relaxation of the mind** Relaxation can take the form of 'time out' to have a rest or a change. Focusing on quiet music, reading a magazine, or chatting to a friend can help a person think more clearly.

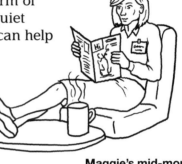

Maggie's mid-morning break

Sleep

Sleep is a state of natural unconsciousness. The amount of sleep needed varies from person to person. It also varies with age. Generally, babies need about 16 hours of sleep a day, whereas adults need much less. Good, sound sleep is essential for health and can be encouraged by:

- physical exercise that tires the body;
- a warm, comfortable bed in a quiet darkened room;
- the ability to put worries aside;
- a warm caffeine-free drink, but no excess alcohol or late TV.

Lack of sleep The body needs sleep to allow the brain to function efficiently. Lack of enough sleep makes people irritable, unable to concentrate, clumsy and more at risk of accidents. Being repeatedly short of sleep can lead to stress that results in anxiety and depression.

12. **a i** What is relaxation,
   ii Why is it helpful in health and care settings,
   iii why is 'time out' useful,
   iv what forms can it take?
   b What happens during relaxation?
   c What actions help relaxation of:
      i the body,
      ii the mind?
   d i What is sleep,
      ii how much sleep is needed,
      iii what encourages sound sleep?
   e Give four effects of lack of sleep.

Activity

Prepare a questionnaire on sleep and use it with friends and family to find the average amount of sleep per night. Are variations in the amount of sleep related to different age groups? (➲ page 246 'Questionnaire'.)

Too much tea or coffee are well known causes of insomnia, palpitations and nervousness.

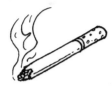

The nicotine in cigarettes is addictive, and other substances in smoke cause cancer.

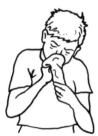

Solvent abuse When inhaled, fumes from solvents such as lighter fuel, glues and cleaning fluid produce feelings of being drunk. The effects come and go quickly, but they can have harmful effects on the body and can be the cause of accidents.

13. a What is substance abuse?
  b What do drugs do?
  c Explain the differences between medicines and illegal drugs.
  d i Name three social drugs.
   ii Give two examples of the effect of social drugs on health.
  e What is drug abuse?
  f Explain why care needs to be taken with all drugs.
  g How does drug addiction differ from drug abuse?
  h Explain the difference between physical and psychological dependence.
  i Who can advise drug addicts?
  j Describe solvent abuse.

Substance abuse

Substance abuse is the misuse of various substances that cause a risk to health such as drugs, solvents and alcohol.

Drugs

Drugs alter the way the body or the mind works.
- **Medicines** are drugs used to treat and prevent disease. Some can be bought over the counter at a pharmacy. Others can only be obtained by prescription from doctors or dentists.
- **Social drugs** are widely used on social occasions and include alcohol, nicotine in cigarettes and caffeine in tea and coffee.
- **Illegal drugs** are drugs that have been banned by law for use in this country, and it is illegal to possess or supply them. They include cannabis, heroin, cocaine, crack, ecstasy and LSD.

Drug abuse (drug misuse)

Drug abuse occurs when drugs are used for the wrong reasons. Care needs to be taken with all drugs, including medicines, because they have side effects that can cause long-lasting harm if misused or taken in excess of the recommended dose. They:
- have different effects on different people;
- are dangerous if taken in the wrong doses;
- can be addictive, for example alcohol, nicotine, heroin, crack.

Drug addiction (drug dependence)

Drug addiction is uncontrolled craving for drugs due to:
- **physical dependence** occurs when the body has become so used to a drug that withdrawal symptoms occur when the supply is cut off, for example pain, nausea, sweating, agitation and depression;
- **psychological dependence** – drugs are taken to make the user 'feel good'. When this feeling wears off, it is replaced by the craving for more of the drug.

Drug treatment

It is much easier to become addicted to drugs than to give them up, but for users who want to kick the habit:
- GPs (family doctors) can give advice, and also refer patients for specialist treatment;
- the National Drugs Helpline gives a free confidential telephone helpline - 0800 776600;
- drug addiction clinics give advice and support.

Activity
Obtain information from two organisations that offer help for drug addicts. Summarise the information from each organisation. Compare the support that they offer.

Smoking

Why tobacco smoke is dangerous to health

Tobacco smoke is a harmful mixture of gases, tar droplets and particles of ash including:

- nicotine - a fast-acting drug that can easily become addictive;
- tar – the sticky brown substance that stains fingers and teeth and contains chemicals that cause cancer;
- carbon monoxide – a poisonous gas.

Every time a smoker inhales, smoke is drawn through the mouth and into the lungs and . . .

. . . nicotine and carbon monoxide pass from the air in the lungs and into the blood. Within a minute, they have travelled in the blood stream to all parts of the body.

. . . tar droplets and ash stick to and coat the sides of the air tubes.

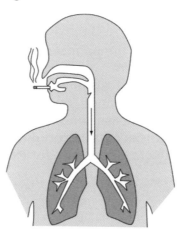

. . . the smoke irritates the mucous membrane that lines the air tubes, causing increased amounts of mucus (phlegm) to be produced. The mucus builds up and blocks the air tubes. Coughing, especially first thing in the morning, removes some of the mucus.

Mucus builds up in the lungs and becomes infected. **Pus** from the infection causes bad breath.

Diseases linked with smoking

Smoking day after day, year after year, puts increasing strain on the body and makes a smoker more prone to diseases such as:

- **cancer** of the mouth, larynx, oesophagus, lung and bladder;
- **lung diseases** – bronchitis, emphysema and pneumonia;
- **blocked arteries** – these interfere with the blood supply and are the cause of heart attacks and strokes, gangrene and the possible amputation of the toes, feet or legs.

Smoking and pregnancy

When a pregnant mother smokes, substances in the smoke such as nicotine and carbon monoxide pass from the mother's blood into the baby's bloodstream and affect the baby's health. Pregnant women who smoke are more likely to have:

- a miscarriage;
- a still-born baby, or one who dies in the first week after birth;
- a smaller, weaker baby;
- a baby who suffers from lung infections.

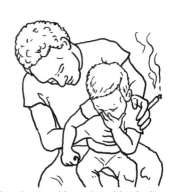

Passive smoking – breathing in the smoke from other people's cigarettes – increases a non-smoker's risk of lung cancer. Also the children of smokers suffer more from asthma, bronchitis, pneumonia and other chest infections.

Activity

Produce a poster to warn children against smoking.

---

14. a Explain why tobacco smoke is dangerous to health.
  b Describe what happens every time smoke is inhaled.
  c Name three diseases linked with smoking.
  d How do substances in smoke reach unborn babies?
  e When pregnant women smoke, name four effects that it can have on their babies.

Alcohol

When a person drinks alcohol, it is absorbed into the blood stream from the stomach and small intestine. It is absorbed more quickly from an empty stomach than from one containing food. The alcohol travels in the blood stream and reaches all parts of the body. It continues to circulate until it has been destroyed in the liver, or leaves the body in breath or urine.

Effects on the brain

Alcohol is a sedative and slows down the activity of the brain. It:

- numbs the pain centre, making the drinker less aware of discomfort;
- reduces restraints on behaviour, making it easier to relax, talk and laugh loudly;
- may release sentimental or aggressive feelings;
- reduces muscle coordination, resulting in unsteadiness;
- affects judgement, for example when driving a car.

Activity

Produce a poster showing:
i   the government guidelines on alcohol intake for males and females;
ii how many units of alcohol are contained in drinks ordered at a bar;
iii the legal alcohol limits for drivers.

Effects on the body

Brain (see above).

Eyes have difficulty in focusing.

Speech is slurred.

Hands become unsteady.

Legs become unsteady.

Stomach – too much alcohol irritates the stomach wall causing nausea (feeling sick) and vomiting (being sick).

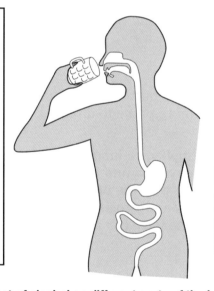

Removal of alcohol from the body

Liver – alcohol circulates around the body until the liver has had time to destroy it.

Lungs breathe out a little alcohol.

Kidneys excrete a little alcohol in urine.

Effect of alcohol on different parts of the body

15. a When a person drinks alcohol:
    i   how does it reach the brain,
    ii how long does it stay in the body?
  b Why is alcohol a sedative?
  c Why does alcohol:
    i   ease aches and pains,
    ii make talking easier,
    iii make some people want to fight,
    iv cause clumsiness,
    v   increase car accidents,
    vi cause vomiting?
  d What effect can alcohol have on:
    i   the eyes,
    ii speech,
    iii the legs?

Social problems caused by alcohol

Heavy drinking can result in a number of social problems.

- **Antisocial behaviour** Alcohol reduces a person's control over their behaviour. It can result in vandalism, fighting, vomiting or urinating in the street. Wife-beating, baby-battering and rape are more common following a drinking session.
- **Absenteeism** A heavy drinker may be too ill to go to work, be late for work, or not be able to work properly. It is easy for such people to lose their jobs.
- **Unhappy homes** One person with an alcohol problem affects the whole family with their unpredictable behaviour.
- **Unprotected sex** Drunkenness that leads to casual sex can also result in pregnancy and the spread of sexual infections.
- **Drink-driving offences** Even small amounts of alcohol increase the dangers of accidents because judgement is impaired and reaction times are slower.

Health problems caused by alcohol

- **Gastritis** Alcohol irritates the inside of the stomach, which becomes inflamed and causes nausea (feeling sick), vomiting (being sick), and loss of appetite.
- **Malnutrition** Because large quantities of alcohol reduce the appetite, heavy drinkers tend not to have a balanced diet. Although they get enough calories from alcohol, they may suffer from lack of vitamins.
- **Cirrhosis of the liver** Large and regular amounts of alcohol gradually destroy the liver.
- **Effects on the brain** Alcohol eventually destroys the brain cells of heavy drinkers, resulting in loss of memory, personality changes and reduced personal care.
- **Alcoholism** is an addiction that occurs when a person cannot control his or her drinking and drinks to excess. Alcoholics usually deny that they have a problem.
- **Fetal alcohol syndrome** This occurs when the mother's heavy drinking poisons her unborn baby. The result is low birthweight, retarded growth and other abnormalities.

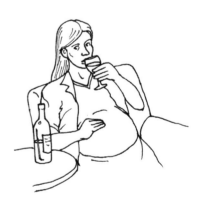

16. **a** Why may heavy drinking result in:
- **i** antisocial behaviour
- **ii** absenteeism
- **iii** unhappy homes
- **iv** unprotected sex
- **v** drink-driving offences?

b Describe the alcohol-related illness:
- **i** gastritis
- **ii** cirrhosis of the liver
- **iii** malnutrition
- **iv** effects on the brain
- **v** alcoholism
- **vi** fetal alcohol syndrome.

Activity

Access the website for Alcoholics Anonymous and Al-Anon to find out:
- **i** the purpose of the organisations,
- **ii** who can become a member,
- **iii** what is the difference between open and closed meetings?

Sexual health

Sexual intercourse (sex) is a natural human activity, and the survival of the human race depends on it. It can result in:

- happiness and contentment, or distress;
- pregnancy if contraception is not used – this is good news if a baby is wanted, but bad news if a baby is unwanted;
- catching a sexually transmitted infection.

Problems of unprotected sex

Unprotected sex occurs when no condoms are used to prevent pregnancy or a sexual infection. Research shows that people are having an increasing number of sexual partners and often having sex at a younger age. This has resulted in increasing numbers of:

- teenage pregnancies;
- women at risk of becoming infertile;
- the spread of sexually transmitted infections.

Sexually transmitted infections (STIs)

A number of microbes (germs) can infect the sex organs and cause infection. These infections can pass from one person to another during sexual contact and cause a variety of problems. For example:

- **chlamydia** can make women infertile;
- **genital herpes** causes highly infectious sores;
- **genital warts** increase the risk in women of developing cervical cancer;
- **gonorrhoea** causes irritation and discharge from the vagina or penis;
- **syphilis** is dangerous if not treated;
- **hepatitis B** is a type of jaundice that can also be spread by dirty needles that are used to inject drugs - a vaccine is now available for those at risk of infection;
- **HIV** (human immunodeficiency virus) spreads through contact with blood or with the sexual fluid in the vagina of females or from the penis in males.

Sexual health clinics (GUM clinics for Genito-Urinary Medicine; STI clinics)
These are NHS clinics for all aspects of sexual health. For example, they give free, confidential advice and treatment to people who think they may have an STI, or need contraceptive advice, or have problems with the loss of sex drive or erections.

17. a Name two unwanted results of sexual intercourse.
- **b i** What is unprotected sex,
- **ii** what has research shown,
- **iii** what has resulted?
- **c i** What is an STI?
- **ii** Describe the effects of seven STIs.
- **d** What is the purpose of sexual health clinics?
- **e** What is the meaning of GUM?

Activity

Find out where the clinics dealing with sexual health are situated in your area. Mark them on the street map of your area. (➲ Activity page 4.)

Abuse

Abuse is the deliberate ill-treatment of other people. It happens in all sections of society and can be:

- **physical** – hitting, punching, cigarette burns, kicking or handling people roughly when assisting them;
- **emotional (psychological)** – the victim's feelings are hurt and their self-esteem damaged by being shouted at (verbal abuse), bullied, wrongly blamed, humiliated or isolated;
- **neglect** – persistent failure to provide food, clothes, warmth, comfort or medical care;
- **sexual** – ranging from sexual remarks and unwelcome touching of the sexual areas of the victim to sexual assault and rape;
- **financial** – theft of money, fraud (cheating victims out of money or possessions), or putting pressure on the victim to give the abuser money, or make a will in the abuser's favour.

Individuals most likely to be at risk Abuse happens to people who are weaker than their abusers and cannot defend themselves. Those most at risk are children, people who have learning difficulties, those who are disabled or have mental health problems, elderly people, and women suffering domestic violence. Abuse can have long-term damaging effects such as depression and low self-esteem.

Domestic violence

Domestic violence is abuse within a relationship and is an illegal offence. It is carried out by people of varying age, race, class, culture or religion, and often follows heavy drinking. In most cases it takes place in the home with a man attacking a woman. Options for those suffering domestic violence include remaining in their own homes with personal alarms linked to the police, spending time in temporary accommodation or a **refuge** (a hostel that provides emergency accommodation, protection and support), being re-housed, or a legal separation or divorce.

Elder abuse

Elder abuse is the deliberate ill-treatment of elderly people and it can occur in any, or all, of the five ways listed above. Giving long-term care to people when they are ill, in pain, depressed, forgetful, ungrateful or abusive can be very demanding and exhausting. When an elderly person is abused by relatives who are 'at the end of their tether', the abused person needs protection and their carers need help and support.

18. **a** What is abuse?
    b Describe five types of abuse.
    c Who are most at risk from abuse?
    d i What is domestic violence?
      ii where does it usually take place,
      iii what sort of people are involved?
    e Give five options to avoid domestic violence.
    f i What is elder abuse,
      ii when may carers become exhausted,
      iii who needs protection,
      iv who needs support?

Activity

Find out about child abuse. For example from *Child Care & Development* by Pamela Minett.

Protection from abuse

Helping to protect individuals from abuse includes:

- raising awareness of the problem;
- noting and recording any signs of possible abuse such as bruises, burns, scalds, or changes in behaviour - the victim could be frightened, or depressed, have difficulties in sleeping or be off their food;
- training staff so that they are aware of the procedures to follow when incidents are reported to them.

Positive vetting

Only adults who have been positively vetted by the CRB (Criminal Records Bureau) are considered safe to work with children and vulnerable adults (elderly and disabled people). If there is any evidence that they pose a risk of causing harm they are barred.

Self harm

Self harm occurs when individuals deliberately harm themselves. This can take a number of forms including:

- cutting the skin;
- punching oneself;
- burning oneself;
- throwing the body against something hard;
- pulling out hair;
- scratching, picking or tearing at one's skin causing sores and scarring;
- starving (anorexia);
- bulimia (self-induced vomiting);
- taking an overdose of medicines.

Why people self-harm

Some people self-harm when they are unable to cope with a specific problem, and they stop once the problem is resolved. Others self-harm whenever certain pressures or feelings arise. It may happen on a regular basis, or just once or occasionally. A few people who self-harm attempt to kill themselves (suicide). This may not be a serious attempt to escape from life but a desperate 'cry' for help.

Activity

An individual who is addicted to drugs will need medical help and counselling. A number of factors that influence health have been discussed in this section. Identify four factors and explain:

i   the effects the addiction can have on the health of the individual;
ii how the problems of the addicted individual can then affect their care needs.

19. a What signs of abuse should be recorded?
    b Name two other actions that help protect from abuse.
    c i Who must be positively vetted,
       ii what does positive vetting mean?
    d In what ways do people harm themselves?
    e Why do people self-harm?
    f Give an explanation for attempted suicide.

Health action plan

The object of a health action plan is to work out a plan designed to improve the health of a chosen individual.

1. **Select** a person who wishes to change an aspect of their life that could improve their health, for example:

   - lose weight;
   - gain weight;
   - give up smoking;
   - become more mobile.

2. **Explain** the reasons behind the wish to improve their health.

3. **Assessment** – describe the specific health needs, for example how much weight does the person need to lose or in what ways does mobility need to be increased?

4. **Set targets** in cooperation with the person concerned for:

   - short-term goals, e.g. 1-3 months;
   - medium-term goals, e.g. 3-6 months;
   - long-term goals, e.g. 9 months or more.

5. **Outcome** – describe factors that could affect the outcome and explain why the targets may not be achieved, for example:

   - financial factors;
   - time constraints;
   - social factors.

6. **Identify** the possible effects on health of achieving the targets.

7. **Identify** any risks to health.

8. **Choose** a day to start the plan.

9. **Monitor** progress at regular intervals.

10. **Outcome** – reflect on the success or otherwise of the health action plan:

    - Was the plan realistic and achievable?
    - Were the targets completed? If not, why not?

Activities

1. Produce an action plan to improve your own health or the health of someone you know well and who is happy to cooperate with you.
2. Describe the factors that may influence an individual's ability to keep to the action plan.
3. Explain the potential physical, social and emotional effects on the individual achieving the targets in the action plan.

Hazards in health and social care environments

Hazards and risks

A **hazard** can be any item, piece of equipment, chemical, biological or radiation agent that has the potential to cause harm.

Risk is the likelihood that a hazard will cause harm.

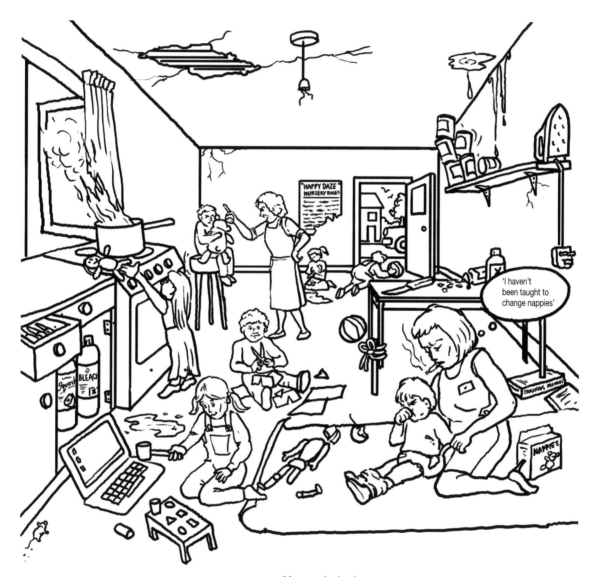

Hazards indoors

Activity

1. **a** Explain the difference between a hazard and a risk.
   b Identify at least 25 hazards in the picture above. List them in the table, add a potential risk and the action needed to avoid/reduce the risk.

Hazard	Risk	Action
Water on the floor		

Hazards outside

Outdoor play areas

It is estimated that there are approximately 40,000 injuries to children in playgrounds each year that result in a hospital visit. Playground accidents are more likely to happen when:

- the playground and equipment are badly maintained;
- the equipment is misused;
- unsuitable clothes and footwear are worn;
- young children lack supervision;
- the equipment lacks rubber matting underneath it to reduce damage to children from the inevitable falls.

Activity

Discuss accidents outside the home and what can be done to prevent them. (➲ page 243 'Discussion'.)

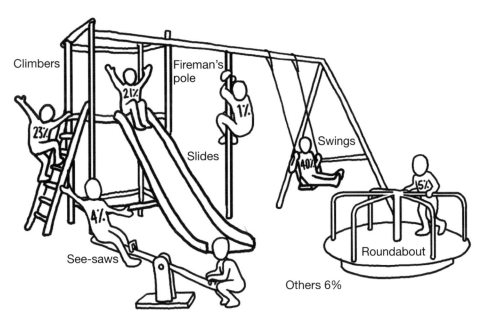

Play equipment involved in falls

Total number of recorded accidents outside the home in one year in England and Wales					
Age in years					
Location	**0-4**	**5-14**	**15-64**	**64-75**	**75+**
Garden/grass/flower beds	1843	3527	6827	1219	1165
Yard/driveway/paths	628	1164	3081	618	670
Patio/terrace/veranda	159	146	440	91	83
Outdoor stairs/steps	158	119	813	133	179
Garage	38	114	912	156	98
Greenhouse	1	0	31	14	15
Sheds/outbuildings	21	8	259	50	37

Data from HASS (Home and Leisure Accident Surveillance System)

2. **a** When are accidents in playgrounds more likely to happen?
   b How many children injured in playgrounds are taken to hospital in a year?
   c List the play equipment in the order in which each is involved in falls, starting with the highest percentage.
   d i Suggest two risks for each of the accidents outside the home.
   ii Suggest a reason why more accidents are recorded for the 15-64 age group than for any other group.

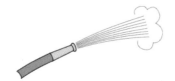

Water cools the burning material. It can be used for solids like wood or paper, but never on electrical fires or burning fat or oil – it makes them worse.

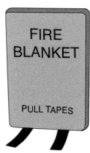

Fire blankets are used to smother flames such as chip pan fires, or for wrapping round someone whose clothing is on fire.

3. **a** Why should fire doors be kept closed at all times?
   b What should happen if a fire occurs?
   c Why is it safest to escape from a fire by crawling?
   d Name five things used for putting out fires.
   e What are the fire safety requirements in health and social care settings?
   f Describe the colour coding for the fire extinguishers.
   g i Why is cool water applied to burns?
   ii What should not be applied to burns?
   iii What action is necessary for large burns?

Fire

A **fire** occurs when something burns and gets out of control. Things to remember about fires include:

- keep fire doors closed at all times to prevent fire from spreading;
- if a fire occurs keep doors and windows shut to contain the flames and stop air from entering (fires need oxygen);
- hot air and smoke rise, so the safest way to escape from a fire is by crawling on the floor;
- there are a number of ways of putting out fires, but no single type of extinguisher is totally effective on every kind of fire.

Emergency first aid for burns Cool in running water for at least 10 minutes to reduce the pain and tissue damage. Cover with moist, sterile gauze or an unused plastic bag. If the burn is large or severe take the patient to a GP or hospital straight away. Do not remove burnt clothing and do not apply creams, butter or oils.

Fire safety

All health and social care settings should have:

- unlocked and unblocked means of escape;
- direction signs to the exits and fire escapes;
- fire extinguishers available;
- fire extinguishers always placed next to the emergency exits;
- fire extinguishers regularly serviced;
- new employees trained in fire drill;
- regular fire drills for all staff.

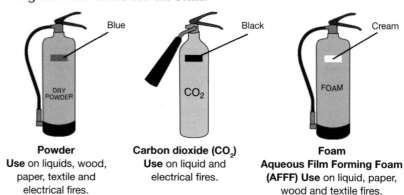

Powder
Use on liquids, wood, paper, textile and electrical fires.

Carbon dioxide (CO$_2$)
Use on liquid and electrical fires.

Foam
Aqueous Film Forming Foam (AFFF) Use on liquid, paper, wood and textile fires.

Types of fire extinguisher

Activities

1. For each of the different types of fire extinguisher, explain its purpose. Give your answer in two columns.
2. In your placement organisation make a note of the position of fire extinguishers and the type being used.

Control of infectious diseases

Infectious diseases are caused by germs that spread from one person to another. Germs are mainly bacteria and viruses and they can spread in several ways by:

- **contact** either by touching an infected person or by handling an object that has picked up the germs – **contagious diseases** are diseases spread by contact;
- **infected droplets** that have been coughed or breathed out;
- **contaminated food and drink** that causes food poisoning;
- **dust** – some germs can survive for a long time in dust and dirt;
- **unsterilised equipment** such as medical instruments and syringes.

Notifiable diseases are diseases that must be reported to the Health Authorities so that they can be rapidly controlled. They include diphtheria, dysentery, food poisoning, hepatitis, malaria, measles, poliomyelitis, tuberculosis, typhoid and whooping cough.

Where infection spreads easily

Infectious disease can spread easily when people are in close contact with each other as happens in residential homes, hospitals, day nurseries and schools. In addition:

- sick and elderly people have lower levels of immunity;
- the immune systems of babies and young children are not yet fully developed.

Reducing the risk of infection

- **Cleanliness (hygiene)** reduces germs.
- **Vaccination** of people most at risk of catching infections. For example, the immunisation programme for children prevents the spread of common childhood diseases, and flu vaccines are offered each year to people most at risk of developing complications such as diabetics and elderly people.
- **Education** of carers, clients and patients on how to avoid infection by actions such as thorough handwashing.

Clean hands
- short, clean nails
- careful hand washing
- cover cuts and grazes with a waterproof plaster

Disposable gloves must be thrown away after use.

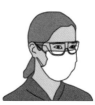

Use face masks and eye protection if there is a risk of fluids splashing into the carer's face.

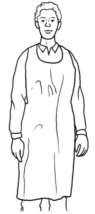

Use disposable aprons if there is a risk of body fluids or blood splashing the carer's clothes.

Ways of protecting against infection

4. **a** What causes infectious diseases?
   b **i** What are contagious diseases?
      ii Name four other ways that diseases can spread.
   c **i** What are notifiable diseases?
      ii Give some examples.
   d **i** When can infectious diseases spread easily,
      ii why are sick and elderly people vulnerable to infection,
      iii why can infections spread easily in day nurseries?
   e Describe three ways of reducing the risk of infection.
   f Describe four ways of protecting against infection.

Activity

Survey a health and social care environment, school or college:
a Identify any potential hazards.
b Describe actions taken to reduce the risks.
c Explain the strengths and weaknesses of actions taken to minimise the risks.

Health and safety legislation and guidelines

Accidents and ill health can ruin people's lives. Not only do they harm the victims but may also affect employers and other workers. A number of laws are in place to promote health and safety in the workplace, and these are therefore important in health and care settings.

Health and Safety at Work Act 1974

This act regulates the health and safety of employees in the workplace. Under this act:

employers are legally required to ensure that the workplace is as safe as possible - safe machinery and equipment, safe working practices, employees trained in safety, protective clothing provided, and an Accidents Book kept.

employees must take care of their own and other's safety at work by following health and safety instructions, using protective clothing and equipment as required, reporting hazards or work-related injuries, and cooperating with their employer on health and safety issues.

Risk assessment

The 'Management of Health and Safety at Work Regulations 1999' requires employers to carry out a **risk assessment** for every work activity. In care settings, this involves identifying hazards and potential risks to service users and their carers. Five steps to assessing risks in the workplace are:

Step 1 Identify the hazards;
Step 2 Evaluate the likelihood of harm occurring;
Step 3 Decide whether the existing control measures are adequate;
Step 4 Record your findings and implement them;
Step 5 Review your assessment and update if necessary.

---

1. a Name three groups of people who are affected when accidents happen at work.
 b To ensure safety in the workplace, what should:
   i the employers do,
   ii the employees do?
 c i Who are required to carry out risk assessments,
   ii what does this involve in care settings?
 d List five steps to assessing risks.

Control of Substances Hazardous to Health Regulations (COSHH) 2002

Using chemicals or other hazardous substances at work can put people at a health risk. For this reason, the law requires employers to control exposure to hazardous substances to prevent ill health.

Types of hazardous substances are:

- materials handled in work activities;
- dust produced by work activities;
- fumes produced during work activities;
- radioactive materials;
- biological waste that could contain germs.

Effects of hazardous substances on health include:

- skin irritation or dermatitis as a result of skin contact;
- asthma as a result of contact with substances at work;
- losing consciousness due to inhaling toxic fumes;
- cancer, which may appear long after the exposure to the chemicals or radiation that caused it;
- infection from bacteria and other germs;
- poisoning from ingesting toxic substances.

Hazard signs

International hazard signs are produced in different colours:

R – red means that an action is forbidden;
B – blue means action must be taken;
Y – yellow warns of potential danger;
G – green gives information.

Risk of harm

Flammable

Hand protection

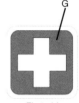
First aid

Toxic

Biological hazard

Ear protection

No naked flames

Corrosive

Prohibited for drinking

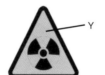
Radiation risk

Eye protection

> ## Activity
>
> Design a safety poster to display in a health and care setting.

2. **a** Why is a law needed to control exposure to hazardous substances?
   b Link each type of hazardous substance with an effect on health. Give your answers in a table.
   c Describe the colour coding of hazard signs.
   d Draw and colour three signs that show actions that must be taken.
   e Draw and colour the sign that:
      i warns of the risk of harm,
      ii shows an action that is prohibited,
      iii warns of radiation,
      iv gives information.
   f Draw and colour a sign that warns that a substance:
      i is liable to catch fire,
      ii is poisonous,
      iii could eat away substances,
      iv could contain germs?

Manual Handling Operations Regulations 1992

Manual handling includes lifting, putting down, pushing, pulling, carrying or moving objects or people. These actions are responsible for about half the injuries in the health and care services. Many are back injuries and lead to, on average, 20 days off work. In some cases the victim never recovers. Other injuries arise from repetitive movements or difficult-to-handle loads. Injuries are far more likely to arise when employees:

- are physically unsuited to carry out the task;
- are wearing unsuitable clothing or footwear;
- do not have adequate training.

Regulations were brought in to reduce the number of injuries caused by manual handling. They require:

- **employers** to avoid the need for hazardous manual handling as far as reasonably practicable.
- **employees** to be responsible for following any systems of work that have been laid down to avoid potential injury, make proper use of equipment provided for their safety, and co-operate with their employer on health and safety matters.

The right way to lift a heavy object

1. Hold the heaviest part of the object closest to the body.
2. At the time of lifting, tighten the abdominal muscles; this reduces the strain on the back.
3. When lifting, push up with the muscles of the legs.

Reporting of Injuries, Diseases and Dangerous Occurrences Regulations (RIDDOR)

Employers, self-employed people and those in control of work premises are required to report work-related accidents, diseases and dangerous occurrences. The information enables the Health and Safety Executive (HSE) and local authorities (referred to as 'the enforcing authorities') to identify where and how risks arise and to investigate serious accidents. They are then able to advise on how to reduce injury, ill health and accidental loss.

Activities

1. Describe the main principles of health and safety legislation and guidelines for health and social care environments.
2. Produce a leaflet to explain the main principles of health and safety legislation and guidelines for health and social care environments.

3. a What does manual handling mean?
   b i Describe the injuries caused by manual handling,
     ii when are they more likely to arise?
   c i Why were regulations for manual handling needed,
     ii what do they require from employers,
     iii what three things do they require from employees?
   d Describe the right way to lift a heavy object.
   e What does RIDDOR mean and who does it apply to?

Chapter 3
Vocational Experience

This chapter covers:

- Completing the application process for a period of work experience in a health or social care setting.

- Completing a period of work experience in a health or social care setting.

- Demonstrating the use of interpersonal skills in work experience.

- Describing a period of work experience in a health and social care setting.

Work Experience

Work experience is time in a place of work learning about a particular job or area of work. It may be a **full-time placement** for between 1 and 4 weeks, usually for the same hours as other people who work there, or an **extended work placement** for one day a week over several months.

Work experience gives you an opportunity to:

- get an insight into the world of work;
- find out what skills employers are looking for;
- meet a variety of people and develop interpersonal and communication skills;
- put into practice the theory learned in the classroom;
- find out if you like that kind of work.

Finding a placement

Work experience in a care setting is a required part of many health and social care courses. If a placement is not arranged by your tutor or teacher, you need to learn the whereabouts of appropriate organisations and care settings. You may find out about them from friends, the job centre, local papers or the internet. You may then wish to apply directly to an organisation that interests you and ask them if they can provide a placement.

Making contact

There are different ways of applying for work experience. You may need to:
- send a CV with a covering letter;
- fill in an application form;
- apply online using an electronic application form;
- make contact by telephone.

Telephone skills

- Plan what you want to say before you make a telephone call and write it down.
- Make the call away from noise and distractions.
- Speak more slowly than you normally would and be polite.
- Introduce yourself clearly, using your first name and surname.
- Keep a record of who you spoke to and what you discussed.
- Any follow-up action that you promised to take should be prompt.

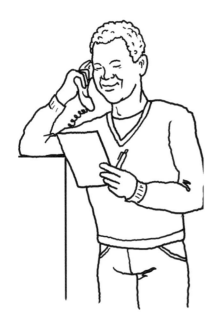

Activity

With a partner, role-play making telephone calls to ask about a placement. Comment on each other's telephone skills.
(Role play ➲ page 244.)

CV (Curriculum Vitae)

Curriculum vitae is Latin meaning 'course of life'. A CV required for work study is an outline of a person's educational and professional history. Items to include are:

- **personal details** – names, address, telephone number and email address;
- **education** – the secondary schools or colleges that you have attended, with dates;
- **qualifications** such as GCSEs or a First Aid Certificate;
- **skills** relevant to the placement, such as computer skills and the level of skill attained;
- **experience** in health and care settings, for example, helping to care for a sick relative, baby-sitting or voluntary work;
- **interests/spare time activities** that would make you suitable for working in a health and care setting, for example an interest in nursing, childcare, or working with older people;
- **two referees** – one should be from your teacher, tutor or employer, the other from someone else who knows you well. It is important to ask permission from people before you name them as referees.

Points to note when writing a CV

It pays to:

- make a rough draft first;
- be honest - don't exaggerate or make things up;
- keep to the facts -only include relevant details;
- leave space around the edges of the page;
- leave a space between each paragraph;
- double check your spelling and grammar;
- if hand-written, ensure that the writing is legible (easy to read).

Application forms

An application form is designed to bring out the essential information and personal qualities that the employer requires. Some employers send out application forms by post. Others have electronic application forms on the internet and require them to be filled in on screen.

Activities

1. Write your own CV using the 'points to note' as a guide.
2. Complete a sample application form. Your tutor can provide you with a sample application form to complete.

Writing letters

People write letters for someone else to read. Whether they are written by hand or using a computer, the information needs to be set out clearly and easy to understand.

- When applying for a placement it is often necessary to write a covering letter and a CV. If you have written your CV on a computer, attach a neat hand-written letter. This demonstrates your computer skills and also your hand-writing.
- When you have been offered a placement it is important to write another letter promptly to say whether you are accepting or declining the offer.

Covering letter for a CV

Your address ....
....
Postcode
Telephone number
Email address

Name of person/organisation you are writing to
Job title
Organisation
Address of the organisation.................
....Post code

Date

Dear Mr/Mrs/Ms ....(if you know the name of the person you are writing to) or
Dear Sir/Madam (If you don't know the name of the person you are writing to)

Say what you are writing to ask for (what kind of work experience).
Say why you need work experience (name the course that you are studying).
Give the amount of time that you are required to carry out work experience.
Personal details - your age, and where you are studying.
Say that a CV is enclosed (and remember to enclose it).

Yours sincerely

Sign the letter with a pen and print your name underneath.

Letters of acceptance or decline

All business letters use a similar format to the one above. The difference between letters is the subject that you are writing about.

- **When you accept a placement:**
  Thank you for your letter dated dd/mm/yy offering me work experience for .... weeks/days, starting on .... (date). I am pleased to accept your offer.

- **When you are not accepting a placement:**
  Thank you for your letter dated dd/mm/yy offering me work experience for .... weeks/days, starting on .... (date). I am grateful for your offer but I am unable to accept it because .... I apologise for any inconvenience that this has caused you.

Activity

Write a letter to accompany your CV asking for a placement at 'The Elms Nursing Home'.

Interview skills

Preparing for the interview

- Most employers expect you to have found out about their organisation and the work they do from, for example, their website or brochure.
- **Dress appropriately** – neat and clean and sensibly.
- **Aim to arrive for the interview early** – plan your journey so that you do not arrive late or flustered.
- **Switch off your mobile**.
- **Prepare questions to ask** – at least three, for example:
  'What sort of work will I be doing?'
  'Do students wear a uniform?'
  'Is there anything I can do to prepare for a placement here?'
- **Shake hands firmly** when you meet the person who is to interview you.

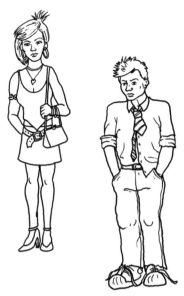

Appearance reflects attitude

During the interview

Questions you might be asked		How to conduct yourself
'Tell me about yourself?'		Look at the interviewer when you are speaking and speak slowly (shows confidence).
'Why do you want work experience here?'	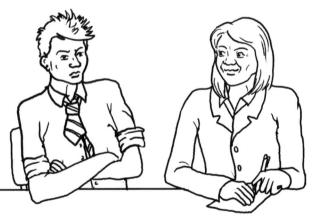	Try to relax, and do not fidget.
'What do you think that working here involves?'		Listen to the questions carefully before answering.
'What do you hope to learn?'		Answer the questions directly, and don't ramble.
'What are your greatest strengths?'		If you haven't understood the question, ask politely for it to be repeated.
'What is your biggest weakness?' 'What are your ambitions in life?'		At the end of the interview, thank the interviewer for seeing you.

Activity

Work with another student to role-play an interview for work experience. Decide who is to be the interviewee and the interviewer. When you have completed the interview, change places and carry out a second interview. Then assess your performance as an interviewee – what did you do well, and what could be improved? (➲ Role play, page 244.)

Using interpersonal skills

Interpersonal skills are the skills used when people relate to each other, and include 'Communication skills' dealt with on pages 6 to 13. These skills are often only noticed when they are absent, for example shouting at clients, ignoring a patient or using a patient's first name without permission.

People with good interpersonal skills are easy to be with. They can relate to other people (and have empathy with them). They know how to deal with feelings that arise in difficult situations instead of being overwhelmed by them.

Using interpersonal skills on work experience

Work experience provides an opportunity to meet a variety of new people. How they treat you will depend partly on the effectiveness of your own interpersonal skills. A person with good interpersonal skills is:

- **non-judgemental** – respects other people's differences of culture, language, race, religion, sexuality and political persuasion.
- **tactful and diplomatic** – being sensitive to other people's feelings and taking the most considerate way to deal with others. Using tact and diplomacy can avoid offence, upset, resentment and opposition.
- **aware of touch or contact**. Some people like to shake hands when they meet you, others do not want to have any bodily contact.
- **aware of personal space** – some service users are uncomfortable when close to others and like to keep some space around them.
- **aware of confidentiality** – do not pass on personal information about a service user without permission.
- **has listening skills** ➲ page 7.

Teamwork skills

Much of the work in health and care settings involves working as part of a team. In addition to using interpersonal skills, a good team member:

- turns up on time;
- is polite, reliable and trustworthy;
- is keen to cooperate with the other team members;
- can follow instructions;
- does not get flustered when under pressure;
- takes responsibility for their own work and behaviour.

Activity

From your work experience placement describe:
a occasions when good interpersonal skills were needed.
b the strengths and weaknesses of your own interpersonal skills.

The Work Experience Report

Keeping a diary or placement log

During work experience, students are required to keep a diary or placement log that describes their daily activities and observations. They will then have the information to make a report of their work experiences. Here are some ideas.

Describe your placement

- Give the name of the organisation.
- State whether it is a statutory, a voluntary, or a private organisation (➲ page 6).
- Identify its purpose - what it does, and what services it supplies.
- Say how it is funded - where the money and other resources come from that enable the organisation to exist, and why they are needed.
- Name the policies you are aware of, for example, in health and safety, data protection or anti-discrimination.
- List any procedures, for example for health and safety, fire evacuation and complaints.
- What are the multicultural factors - the ethnic origin, cultures and religions of the employees and service users, and any special requirements needed for them.

The staff

- **Staffing levels** – is there the right balance of staff (the ideal staff-client ratio) for the number of service users? Are there difficulties in maintaining the right balance to sustain a satisfactory service?
- **Job roles and responsibilities** – list the different types of jobs and the responsibilities involved in each.
- **Skills/qualifications/personal attributes** required for each type of job. Not all jobs require qualifications; personal qualities are sometimes more important.
- **Induction** – the process that all new health and care workers have to undergo when they start.
- **Terms and conditions of employment** – how do staff know about these?
- **Way of monitoring performance**, for example, by appraisal, peer review or client assessment.
- **Opportunities for continuing professional development** – ways that the workforce can improve their skills and knowledge, and gain relevant qualifications.

Activities

1. Using the **Citizens Advice** website, find out about young people and employment:
   i   who is a young worker?
   ii   what are the working hours?
   iii what is the entitlement to rest days and rest breaks?
2. Produce a Health and Safety poster based on information from your placement. Use text, images and data (facts, figures, statistics) on your poster.

Assessment of your own performance

- timekeeping – assess your own record of being on time.
- knowledge gained – what you learnt about working in a caring job.
- skills gained – what you learned to do.
- confidence – how confident you felt.
- initiative – describe occasions when you showed useful initiative.
- activities undertaken – the tasks you were given.
- ability to follow instructions – how well did you do?
- your own strengths – what you have done particularly well.
- your own weaknesses – what you need to improve.
- personal achievements – what did you feel that you had achieved?

Evaluation

- Describe the benefits you gained from work experience.
- Describe the benefits the placement gained from having you there on work experience.

Future employment

- What have you learned from your work experience that could be useful in a career in health and social care?
- Have you any career plans for working in the health and social care sector and, if so, in what area? If not, explain why not.

Activity

Produce a four-page brochure using text, images and data, to describe your placement.

Chapter 4
Cultural Diversity

This chapter covers:

- The diversity of individuals in society.

- Factors that influence the quality of opportunity for individuals in society.

- The practices of different religions and secular beliefs.

- The rights of individuals in health and social care environments.

The diversity of individuals

The diversity of individuals was introduced in Chapter 1 (⮑ pages 14-19). This section further explores diversity and the need for equality of opportunity and individual rights.

The diversity of individuals is the way that people are different from each other due to physical, social and political factors.

- **Physical factors** It is possible to recognise one person from another by how they look. The individual differences in appearance are due to a combination of genes, gender, shape and colour of the face and body, clothing and other differences in appearance.
- **Social factors** involve relationships with people in society, for example family background and marital status.
- **Political factors** involve national and local government policies, for example educational opportunities and welfare benefits.

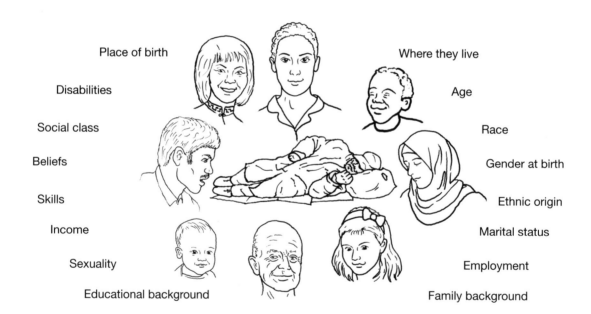

Place of birth
Disabilities
Social class
Beliefs
Skills
Income
Sexuality
Educational background

Where they live
Age
Race
Gender at birth
Ethnic origin
Marital status
Employment
Family background

Social and political factors that make people different from each other

Activity

Compare yourself with another person for each of the social and political factors that make people different from each other. In how many ways are you
i similar, **ii** different?

Ethnicity

An **ethnic group** is a group of people with the same racial origins and cultural traditions. The members of the group may be distinguished by their physical features, common language, or religion. Ethnicity does not relate to the country of birth as members of an ethnic group may be born in any part of the world.

- **'White' (Caucasian)** includes white (light-skinned) British, Europeans, Americans, Australians and New Zealanders.
- **'South Asian'** includes people with ancestral ties to India, Pakistan and Bangladesh.
- **'Black'** includes people from Africa and the Caribbean.
- **'Chinese'** refers to people of the Chinese race; Chinese people are found in many countries throughout the world.
- **'Mixed race'** may be, for example, White/Chinese, Asian/Black, Native American/White or White Australian/Aboriginal.
- Other ethnic groups.

A **census** is an official count of the population in an area that includes personal details such as age, sex, occupation, etc. In the UK, a census of the people and households is carried out every ten years. The 2001 Census asked people which ethnic group they belonged to; the results for England and Wales are shown in the pie chart below.

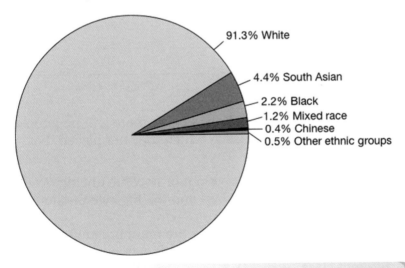

- 91.3% White
- 4.4% South Asian
- 2.2% Black
- 1.2% Mixed race
- 0.4% Chinese
- 0.5% Other ethnic groups

Ethnicity in England and Wales: Census 2001
(UK Population by ethnic group: Social Focus in Brief: Ethnicity)

1. a What is an ethnic group?
   b How may an ethnic group be distinguished?
   c Why is ethnicity not the same as country of birth?
   d Complete the table for five ethnic groups listed above:

Population by Ethnic group in England and Wales: Census 2001		
% of population	Ethnic group	People included in the group

Activity

Find information from the 2001 census about ethnic groups in Scotland or Northern Ireland. Compare the results with the ethnic groups in England and Wales in 2001.

Social class

A **social class** is a group of people who share a common position in society. There used to be three social classes in Britain – upper, middle and lower (working) class. People in these classes had different lifestyles and were recognised by the way they spoke and dressed, their leisure interests, the food they ate, and how they educated their children. Nowadays social class is more commonly linked with occupation. A person's occupation (job) provides the income (money), which in turn affects lifestyle and health.

Class	Occupation
	**Socio-economic Classification for people of working age, National Statistics 2001, England and Wales**
1	Higher managerial and professional occupations:
	1.1 Large employers and higher managerial occupations, e.g. chief executive
	1.2 Higher professional occupations, e.g. doctor, lawyer
2	Lower managerial and professional occupations, e.g. nurse, teacher, policeman
3	Intermediate occupations, e.g. secretaries, firemen, dental nurses, skilled manual
4	Small employers and own account workers, e.g. shopkeepers, hairdressers
5	Lower supervisory and technical occupations, e.g. foreman, plumber
6	Semi-routine occupations, e.g. care assistants, sales assistants, drivers
7	Routine occupations, e.g. waitresses, cleaners, labourers
8	Never worked and long-term unemployed

Whatever type of classification is used, there will be people who do not fit into the class in which they are placed. For example, they may:

- have changed their occupation, or become unemployed;
- have the income of one class and the lifestyle of another class;
- be placed in the same class as the main breadwinner of the family although having the occupation and income of a different class;
- be students doing holiday jobs.

2. **a** What is a social class?
   b i What were the three social classes in Britain,
   ii In what ways did these classes differ?
   c i What is social class linked with these days,
   ii How many classes are there in the 2001 statistics?
   d Give four reasons why statistics based on social class may not be accurate

Family structure

A **family** is a group of individuals who live together and are related by blood, marriage or adoption. It is usual for family members to support each other by helping parents to bring up children, giving advice on problems, providing comfort in times of distress, caring for those who are ill, disabled or old, and some sharing of financial resources.

An **extended family** is a large family group that includes grandparents, parents, children, brothers, sisters, aunts, uncles and cousins. The extended family still exists in many countries and communities, but in industrial and technological societies such as the UK, changes to the traditional family way of life have taken place, and nuclear families are more common.

A **nuclear family** consists of parents and their children. Some of the reasons for the trend towards nuclear families are:

- family members often move away from the family base;
- weakened links between members of an extended family have resulted in other types of family life (➲ page 15);
- effective methods of contraception result in families with fewer children or no children;
- many of the functions of the extended family are now carried out by the health and social care services.

Age

It is easy to be intolerant of people who are a different age but it is useful to remember that:

- everyone grows older (including yourself);
- older people grew up in different conditions from those of today;
- their outlook on life will therefore be different;
- younger people lack experience.

3. **a** What is a family?
   b How can members of a family support each other?
   c What is the difference between an extended family and a nuclear family?
   d Give reasons for the trend towards nuclear families.
   e Give examples of the differences between older and younger people.

Activity

Talk to someone who is much older than you. List the opinions that you share and the topics on which you differ.

Sexuality

Sexuality refers to the way people express the sexual aspects of their lives. It is often also used to refer just to sexual orientation. **Sexual orientation** refers to a person's preference for the type of sexual partner they choose. Most people are **heterosexual** – sexually attracted to people of the opposite sex. A small number are **homosexual** – sexually attracted to people of the same sex; they are sometimes referred to as gay (this applies to both men and women) or as lesbians (applies to women only). **Bisexual** means being sexually attracted to both males and females.

Some people are aware of their sexual orientation from a young age and recognise themselves as heterosexual or homosexual. Others are not so sure. Pressure from the family and attitudes in society and religious groups can cause people to hide their sexual feelings. This can lead to uncertainty, insecurity and fear.

It is easier nowadays than in the past for people to declare that they are homosexual because:

- there is more understanding that sexual feelings can be due to an individual's natural personality;
- there is (or should be) more tolerance of other people's differences;
- legislation has been introduced to prevent discrimination on grounds of sexuality.

Gender

The **gender** of an individual is either male or female. **Gender identity** is the gender to which a person feels he or she belongs. For example when a male undergoes a man-to-woman sex change, his gender identity becomes female.

Gender roles Traditionally in the UK, there were distinct gender roles: women looked after the home and children; the men went to work and were the primary breadwinners. These roles became blurred during the last century because:

- girls were given the same educational opportunities as boys;
- more women joined the workforce;
- many jobs requiring muscle power (manual jobs) that were done by men have disappeared;
- many jobs now use machines or technology that both men and women can operate.

Activity

Design and use a questionnaire to obtain the opinions of a number of people on gender roles. For example:

Do you agree or disagree that:

- there are still distinct gender roles for 'women's work' and 'men's work';
- low-paid or part-time jobs such as cleaning, catering, caring, clerical and shop work are done mainly by women;
- building, farming and the armed forces mainly employ men;
- generally, men reach higher positions and earn more money than women;
- laws are necessary to ensure the equal treatment of men and women?

(➲ page 246 Questionnaires.)

---

4. a What is:
  i sexual orientation,
  ii gender,
  iii gender identity?
  b Explain the difference between heterosexual and homosexual.
  c When does a person become aware of their sexual orientation?
  d Why is life easier for homosexuals these days?

Disabilities

Being **disabled** means being unable to carry out everyday activities, for example being unable to walk, cook a meal, get out of bed unaided, blindness, deafness or learning disabilities. The disability may:

- be present at birth, for example Down's syndrome;
- result from disease, for example dementia;
- be caused by injury, for example a road traffic accident.
- result from normal ageing.

Physical impairment

This is the loss of normal movement for actions such as walking or using the hands. It can be the result of:

- **disease or damage to the nervous system** that affects control and coordination of the muscles, for example cerebral palsy, stroke, multiple sclerosis (MS), Parkinson's disease;
- **damage or disorders affecting bones and joints**, for example fractures or arthritis.

Sensory impairment

This is damage to or a disorder of the sense organs, the nerves or the parts of the brain involved. Sensory impairments include:

- blindness (➲ pages 128-129);
- deafness (➲ pages 130-131);
- speech impediments;
- numbness of the skin.

Mental impairment

Mental impairment is due to damage to the brain that results in difficulties learning, understanding, remembering, using language and sometimes social skills. It can be caused by:

- failure of the brain to develop, for example Down's syndrome;
- brain damage, for example head injury or stroke;
- disease, for example Alzheimers and other dementias.

Long-term illnesses (chronic diseases)

Long-term illnesses include asthma, diabetes and epilepsy. They are disabling when the illness is severe or there are complications.

Activities

1. Talk to people of different age groups. Describe ways in which they are different from you.
2. Take part in a group discussion on the rights of patients/service users (➲ page 21). Use examples to show how understanding peoples' differences enables carers to uphold their rights. An example could be a person with an arthritic hip, a chronic invalid, a teenager with learning difficulties or someone with dementia.

5. a What is meant by being disabled?
   b Give two ways in which people become disabled.
   c i What is physical impairment,
     ii what can it be the result of?
   d i What is sensory impairment?
     ii Give four examples.
   e Give three causes of learning disabilities.
   f i Name three long-term illnesses.
     ii When can they be disabling?

Factors that influence the equality of opportunity for individuals

Equality of opportunity means that everyone should have equal rights to employment and the same access to medical treatment and other services. Although our society generally believes that this is good, there are factors that make it difficult to achieve.

How social and political factors affect equality of opportunity

Ethnicity	People from other countries who cannot read or speak English have a limited choice of jobs, and the language barrier makes access to health and care services difficult.
Religious beliefs	It is illegal for employers to discriminate against employees on grounds of religion unless the demands of the religion make an applicant unsuitable for a particular type of job. For example, a person's dress code may make them unsuitable for a food processing factory, or being prohibited from working on certain days may make shift work difficult.
Social class	People in the lower classes have more long-term illnesses and disabilities than those in other classes. They are often not as well educated and are therefore unable to compete for the better-paid jobs.
Gender	Although men and women should have equal job opportunities, there are jobs that do not have equal appeal to both sexes. For example, women are more attracted to jobs working with young children or as carers or secretaries; men are more attracted to jobs on building sites and as mechanics or lorry drivers. This can mean that women end up working in lower paid jobs.
Sexuality (sexual orientation)	The attitudes of other people towards an individual whose sexual orientation is different can reduce that person's opportunities. Opportunities for employment or promotion can be restricted by a reluctance to employ them, or by failing to accept them on an equal basis.
Family commitments	People who are caring for young children or for old or disabled members of the family may find it impossible to have a paid job. If they do have a job, it is likely to be part-time and with few opportunities for promotion.
Disability	The effects of a disability can often be overcome with the determination of the disabled person and the employers. The effect on equality of opportunity varies greatly according to the type of impairment.
Age	Individuals should be valued for what they can do and not have restrictions placed on them because of their age group.

Activity

For each of the eight factors discussed on this page, give an example of a situation that makes equality of opportunity difficult to achieve. Examples may come from your own experience, or people that you know, or from the media.

Discriminatory practice

Discrimination means the different, often unfair, treatment of a person or group of people. It can be:

- **direct discrimination** when people are treated less favourably because of, for example, gender, race or age.
- **indirect discrimination** when a condition that, though it applies to all, has the effect of putting some people at a disadvantage. For example, members of some religious groups are put at a disadvantage by saying that an applicant for a job must be clean shaven. Indirect discrimination is only allowed when there is a good reason for it, in this example, if a beard is a hygiene risk for the job.

Forms of discrimination

Discrimination can be in the form of prejudice, labelling or stereotyping. It can result in harassment, victimisation or bullying.

Prejudice (prejudging) means judging people before knowing enough about them. It results in an opinion formed before meeting the person (or group of people) and is based on poor information.

Gender   Skin colour

Age   Race

Religion   Disability

Have a different accent   **Excuses for prejudice**   They are foreigners

Social class   Where they live

Hair style   Clothing

Behaviour   Weight

Labelling is a short-cut way of describing or classifying people or things in a word or phrase. Labels given to people are usually intended to be hurtful – such as 'loser', 'no-hoper' or 'stupid'. The label may be an attempt to raise a person's own status by ridiculing someone else, or the person may do as the crowd does in order to remain part of the crowd.

Activity

Collect examples of occasions when you noticed discrimination and suggest how each could be avoided. Discuss your examples with other students.

'Young attractive women wanted for bar work.'

'Call centre rates of pay
Men £8 per hour
Women £7 per hour.'

'Employees must wear the uniform provided of skirts and tee-shirts.'

'Employees applying for promotion must not expect flexible working hours for child care.'

Examples of discrimination

---

2. **a** What is discrimination?
   b Explain the difference between direct and indirect discrimination, giving two examples of each from those above.
   c Name three forms of discrimination.
   d What is prejudice?
   e What excuses may people use for prejudice?
   f i What is labelling,
   ii what is the usual intention,
   iii what may labelling attempt to do?

Stereotyping is putting people into groups based on features that they are assumed to have in common. It is often based on mistrust, fear or suspicion that people in one group have of those in another group.

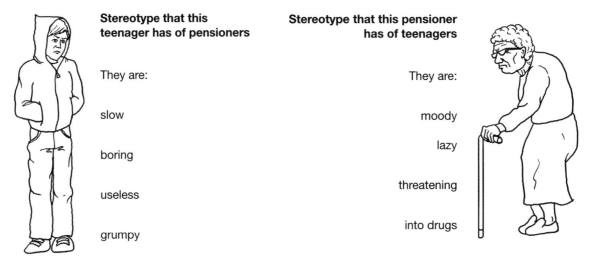

Stereotype that this teenager has of pensioners

They are:

slow

boring

useless

grumpy

Stereotype that this pensioner has of teenagers

They are:

moody

lazy

threatening

into drugs

Harassment means persistent offensive or intimidating behaviour, for example pestering, persecution or abuse which aims to humiliate, undermine or injure its target.

Victimisation means singling somebody out (the victim) for hostile or unfair treatment. For example, when one person is selected out of a crowd to take the blame.

Bullying occurs when one or more people repeatedly intimidate and persecute a weaker person.

Effects of discrimination

When people are treated unfairly it can affect their health and well-being in many ways - physically, socially, emotionally and intellectually. Discrimination can cause people to:

- feel very upset and angry at the unfair treatment;
- lose self-esteem and feel inferior and worthless;
- lose self-confidence in their skills and abilities;
- suffer from worry and depression;
- behave in ways that lead to breakdown of relationships, resulting in loneliness and isolation;
- fail to access or gain the support or help they need from individuals or organisations.

3. a i What is stereotyping,
  ii what is it often based on?
 b in the diagram above
  i what stereotype does the pensioner have of teenagers?
  ii what stereotype does the teenager have of pensioners?
 c Describe:
  i harassment,
  ii victimisation,
  iii bullying.

Activity

Explain the possible effects of discrimination on the physical, intellectual, emotional and social health and well-being of individuals. Your answer can be based on your own experience, that of people you know or examples from the media.

Non-discriminatory practice in health and social care

Because the effects of unfair discrimination can be so severe and long-lasting, it is important for everyone working in the health and social care sectors to treat people fairly and equally.

Responsibilities of individual care workers

Discrimination is prevented when individual care workers:

- are friendly and approachable to everyone – service users, colleagues and supervisors;
- promote equal opportunities;
- follow codes of practice.

Responsibilities of employers

Discrimination is discouraged when employers make clear that they value the different cultures in the workplace. This happens when:

- **diversity is promoted** at all levels from the boss to the new trainees;
- **managers are trained** to get the best out of people from different backgrounds and abilities;
- **information is provided** about the different religions and cultures reflected in the workforce and the customers – when, for example, dates of religious festivals are put on the notice board, and the events are openly displayed, then everyone feels included;
- **a climate of respect is promoted in the workplace** by setting clear standards of behaviour for everyone and by prompt action being taken to deal with any instance of racism, ageism, sexism or religious prejudice;
- **social occasions include everyone** and people do not feel excluded by activities that could upset them, for example those involving alcohol, forbidden foods or gambling;
- **staff are consulted** by regular conversations with management members of their team.

4. **a** Why is it important to treat people fairly?
   b How can health and social care workers prevent discrimination?
   c How can employers discourage discrimination:
   i in the training of managers,
   ii by providing information,
   iii by promoting a climate of respect?

Activity

Colin moves into your care home on the same day as Mary (➲ page 29). Colin is losing his eyesight because of his diabetes. He was a Sergeant Major in the army and he is quite demanding and determined that things will be done his way. However, he is also quite relieved to be moving into the care home because life at home on his own was becoming difficult.

As their carer:
i in what ways will you treat Colin and Mary in the same way?
ii in what ways do you think you will treat Colin and Mary differently?
iii How will you ensure that you treat both Colin and Mary fairly and equally, while respecting their rights and differences.

The role of the media

Books, leaflets, newspapers, magazines, television and the internet help to shape people's opinions.

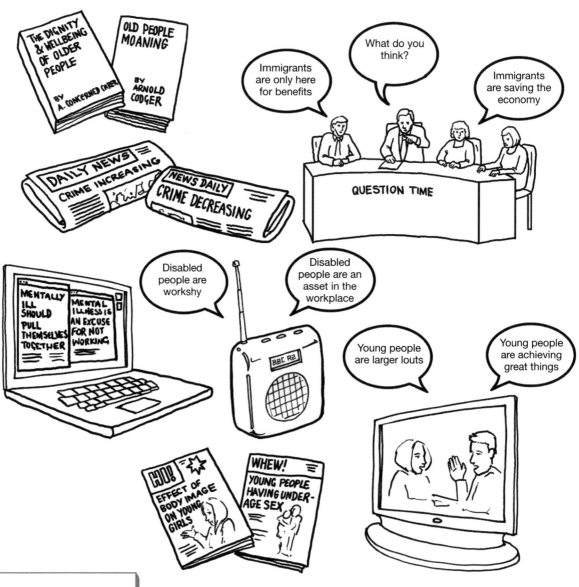

Activity

Find two of your own examples of media stories that you think encourage discrimination. Give a presentation to other students that explains why you think these are examples of discrimination. Also explain what you think could be done by the media to discourage discrimination.

5. a Which opinions on this page do you think encourage or support discrimination and prejudice?
   b Which opinions on this page do you think help to discourage discrimination and reduce prejudice?

Practices in different religious or secular beliefs

Beliefs are thoughts, feelings, attitudes and values that an individual believes to be true. Beliefs may be religious or secular (non-religious) but they are part of an individual's identity. They affect how they live their lives. Beliefs can also lead to intolerance, stereotyping and labelling.

Religion in the UK

Britain is a multi-faith society in which most of the world's religions are practised, with everyone having the right to practise their own religion. All faiths have their own special days when significant events are remembered or celebrated. Health and social care workers will find themselves caring for service users who hold a variety of religious beliefs. All carers should be aware of the customs and requirements of the different religions so that they do not cause offence or distress to their patients or clients.

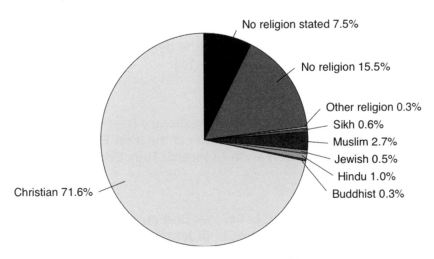

No religion stated 7.5%

No religion 15.5%

Other religion 0.3%
Sikh 0.6%
Muslim 2.7%
Jewish 0.5%
Hindu 1.0%
Buddhist 0.3%

Christian 71.6%

Religion in the UK: Census 2001

As the pie chart above shows, the main religion in the UK is Christianity. There are many different forms of Christianity including Protestants such as The Church of England, The Church of Wales, The Presbyterian Church of Scotland and Methodists. There are also the Roman Catholic Church, the Orthodox Church and a number of other Christian-based religions.

Activity

Find out how many different religions are practised in your nearest town. Mark in the places of worship on a map (➲ page 4 'Activity'). Name each place and the religion that is practised there.

1. **a i** What are beliefs
    ii what do they form part of?
   b What does secular mean?
   c Why can Britain be called a multi-faith society?
   d Name two things that all faiths have.
   e Why is it important for care workers to know about the different religious requirements and customs?
   f List the different religions in the UK, starting with the highest percentage.
   g Name six different forms of Christianity.

World religions

Three of the world's oldest religions all believe in the same God who created everything in the universe. Judaism (the religion of the Jews) is the oldest of these, followed by Christianity (the Christian religion), and Islam (the Muslim religion). All these religions originated in the Middle East.

Christianity

Christianity is based on the teachings of Jesus Christ who lived about 2 000 years ago. Christians believe that God sent his Son, Jesus Christ, to earth to save mankind, and that their lives should be lived according to the love of God.

Christians worship in churches and chapels, their sacred book is the Bible, and their spiritual leaders are called bishops, cardinals, popes, priests or ministers. Sunday is the traditional holy day and day of rest for Christians. Special days of remembrance or celebration include Christmas Day (the birth of Christ), Good Friday (the death of Christ) and Easter Day (the resurrection of Christ).

Care notes

- Most Christians do not have any dietary restrictions although some may wish not to eat meat on Fridays.
- Some Christians may wish to receive Holy Communion.

Judaism

Judaism is based on the belief that God appointed the Jews to be his chosen people in order to set an example of holiness and moral behaviour to the world. Jews worship in synagogues, the Torah is their most important sacred book, and their spiritual leaders are called Rabbis.

The Jewish holy day – the Sabbath – begins at sunset on Friday and lasts until sunset on Saturday. Special days include The Feast of the Passover and The Day of Atonement (Yom Kippur).

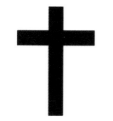

The cross is the symbol of Christianity.

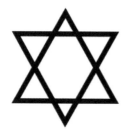

The star of David is the symbol of Judaism.

2. **a** **i** Name two things that Christianity, Judaism and Islam all have in common.
   ii Draw the symbol of each religion.

Care notes

- Orthodox Jews may wish to wash themselves in running water before and after eating.
- Only 'Kosher' food is acceptable to many Jewish people, meaning that it is prepared in accordance with Jewish religious law. Pork and shellfish are prohibited foods.
- Jews usually pray three times a day and privacy and peace should be allowed for this.
- Jews who observe the Sabbath as a day of rest will have limits on what they may do on that day.

Islam

Muslims are followers of the religion of Islam founded about 1 400 years ago. Islam is based on the teachings of Mohammed. The revelations of God (Allah) to Mohammed are written down in the Koran – the holy book of Islam. Muslims worship in mosques, their holy day is Friday, and their preachers are called Imams. There are two divisions of Islam – the Sunnis and the Shia.

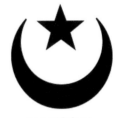

The symbol of Islam (the Muslim religion)

Special days include Eid-ul-Fitr which marks the end of Ramadan - the month during which Muslims fast from sunrise to sunset. The festival of the Hajj – the pilgrimage to Mecca – is known as Eid-ul-Adhia.

Care notes

- Physical examinations should generally be carried out by a doctor or nurse who is the same gender as the patient.
- Permission must be given by the patient/family before jewellery is removed as it often has a special religious significance.
- Many Muslims prefer to wash in running water, so a shower is preferable to a bath.
- Only 'Halal' meat must be eaten, meaning that it is slaughtered in accordance with Muslim religious law. Pork is forbidden.
- Alcohol is forbidden.

3. Compare the three religions by completing the table.

Religion	Christianity	Judaism	Islam
Who founded the religion? Places of worship Holy book Holy day of the week Special days			

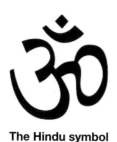

The Hindu symbol

Hinduism

Hinduism originated over 3 000 years ago near the River Indus in modern-day Pakistan. Hindus believe in one eternal God called Brahman, who created and is present in everything. Krishna, Vishnu, Shiva and other gods of the Hindu faith represent different aspects of Brahman. Worship takes place in the home before a shrine or in a Hindu temple.

Hindus believe that the soul passes through a cycle of successive lives and its next incarnation is always dependent on how the previous life was lived. They celebrate many holy days, but the Festival of Lights, Diwali, is the best known.

Care notes

- Hindus generally prefer to be treated and cared for by staff of the same gender.
- Permission must be given by the patient or the family before jewellery is removed as it often has a special religious significance.
- Hindus prefer to shower rather than bathe, and water for washing should be provided when they go to the toilet.
- Most Hindus are vegetarian, refusing to take the lives of animals for food.
- Devout Hindus pray at sunrise, noon and sunset.

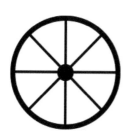

The Buddhist symbol

Buddhism

Buddhism was founded by Buddha about 2 500 years ago in his quest for Enlightenment. It is more a 'way of life' than a religion, and there are many forms. Worship takes place at home or in a temple, with festivals occurring throughout the year. Buddhists pay respects to images of the Buddha but he is not worshipped as a god.

Buddhism focuses on personal spiritual development and strives for deep insight into the true nature of life. It involves meditation as a way of taking control of the mind so that it becomes peaceful and focused.

Care notes

- Most Buddhists are vegetarian.
- Some Buddhists do not drink alcohol and refuse to accept medication that contains alcohol or animal products.

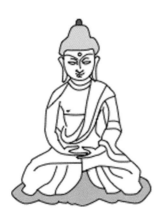

Sikhism

Sikhism was founded about 600 years ago in the Punjab (now a part of India and Pakistan) and is based on the teachings of **Guru Nanak** and other gurus. Sikhs believe in one God who guides and protects them, and that everyone is equal before God. For Sikhs in Britain, the main day to worship in their temples is Sunday. Their main festival is Diwali, the Festival of Light.

The Sikh symbol

Sikhs have five 'signs' of their religion that they should wear at all times. They are:

- uncut hair – Sikhs are not allowed to cut hair from any part of their body (Sikh women are also forbidden to cut any body hair or even trim their eyebrows);
- a wooden comb;
- cotton underwear, not below the knee;
- a steel bracelet worn on the right wrist;
- a short, sheathed ceremonial sword (often in the form of a badge in the UK) – the sword is not worn as a weapon but indicates bravery in defending the faith and protecting the weak.

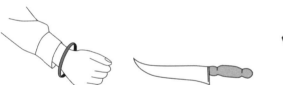

Care notes

- Sikhs generally prefer to be treated and cared for by staff of the same gender, and to remain as covered as possible.
- Removal of any of the 'signs' of their religion must be agreed by the patient or their family.
- Sikhs prefer to use running water for washing and to shower rather than bathe.
- Although there are no rules about not eating meat, many Sikhs are vegetarian.

4. Compare the three religions by completing the table.

Religion	Buddhism	Hinduism	Sikhism
When was it founded? Place of worship Holy day of the week Special days Washing Dietary restrictions			

Jehovah's Witnesses

Jehovah's Witnesses are members of a Christian-based religious movement founded by Charles Taze Russell in the USA towards the end of the 19th century. They believe that:

- God the Father (Jehovah) is 'the only true God';
- the Bible is the Word of God and is historically accurate;
- that humanity is now in its 'last days' and that the final battle between good and evil will happen soon.

Religion occupies much of the time of each Witness, reading and studying their faith on their own and in home groups, and attending meetings in the Kingdom Hall closest to their home. The most important religious event of the year is the commemoration of the Memorial of Christ's Death. Witnesses do not celebrate Christmas, Easter, people's birthdays or have any other festivals.

All Witnesses who are physically able to do it engage in missionary work. They are known for their door-to-door visits offering Bible literature, and recruiting and converting people to what they believe is 'the truth'.

Care notes

- Jehovah's Witnesses refuse blood transfusions, including their own stored blood, even in life-threatening situations.

Rastafari

Rastafarians (Rastas) are members of an African-centred religion that developed in Jamaica after the coronation of Haile Selassie as King of Ethiopia in 1930. They worship Haile Selassie as God and their meetings involve meditation.

Care notes

- Rastafarians generally eat only natural, unpreserved foods, mainly fruit and vegetables. Many avoid milk, meat, shellfish, fish more than 12 inches long, coffee, salt, tobacco and alcohol.
- They are forbidden to cut their hair, so it grows long and is coiled into dreadlocks.

Activity

Chose one of the religions mentioned on pages 77 to 82. Find out more about it, then describe it in a four-minute talk.

---

5. a i Who are Jehovah's Witnesses,
     ii what do they believe in,
     iii where are meetings held,
     iv what is their most important religious event?
   b i What do Jehovah's Witnesses not celebrate,
     ii what medical procedures do they refuse?
   c i Describe the Rastafarian religion.
     ii What rules apply to their hair and their diet?

Secular beliefs

Secular beliefs are those not based on religion or on the worship of God. Atheists and humanists believe that moral values are rooted in our human experience. This life is all we have and that all our efforts should go into making it as enjoyable and satisfying as possible for everyone.

Humanism

Humanists believe that moral values are founded on human nature, rational thinking and experience. Humanism includes atheism and agnosticism. The humanist emblem shows a stylised human figure reaching out to achieve full potential.

Atheism

Atheism denies the existence of all gods. Atheists often have a similar moral code to religious people, but they arrive at the decision of what is good or bad without any help from the idea of god. An **agnostic** believes that it is not possible to know if God exists.

Paganism

Paganism includes a varied collection of beliefs with groups concentrating on specific traditions, practices or elements such as ecology, witchcraft, Celtic traditions or certain gods. Wiccans, Druids, Shamans, Sacred Ecologists, Odinists and Heathens all make up parts of the Pagan community.

Identifying a person's beliefs

Carers should never make assumptions based only on the appearance of service users. Sometimes it is possible to identify a patient or client's personal beliefs by the way they dress. Often this is not possible. The best way to check is to ask them politely if they have any special care needs or preferences.

6. **a** What are secular beliefs?
   b What is humanism?
   c What is the difference between an atheist and an agnostic?
   d Give some examples of pagan beliefs.
   e How can carers know about any care needs that are based on the personal beliefs of patients/service users?

Activity

Compare the beliefs and practices of individuals from two contrasting religious groups or secular beliefs.

Rights of individuals

The rights of individuals are discussed on page 21. This section deals with the laws (rules) that protect these rights. These are found in:

- **Acts of Parliament** – laws made by the UK government;
- **European laws** – laws made by the European Parliament;
- **Codes of practice** for employers and employees – rules made for different areas of employment, which are legally binding.

Conventions, legislation and regulations

Human Rights

European Convention on Human Rights and Fundamental Freedoms 1950.

The Human Rights Act 1998

Citizens of the UK have certain basic human rights, which the government and public authorities are legally obliged to respect.
Everyone has the right to:
- life, liberty, education, security and their own beliefs.
- a private life and a family life
- freedom from discrimination and abuse
- no punishment outside the law.

The Equality and Human Rights Commission 2007

The Equality and Human Rights Commission works to eliminate discrimination, reduce inequality and protect human rights. It can take legal action to enforce the laws.

The Race Relations (Amendment) Act 2000

This Act makes it illegal to discriminate against anyone on the grounds of their colour, race, nationality or ethnic origin.

The Sex Discrimination Act 1975

This Act makes it unlawful to discriminate on the grounds of sex between men and women in the areas of education, employment and the provision of goods and services.

Employment Equality Regulations

Equal Pay Act 1970

Employment Equality Regulations:
   (Sexual Orientation) 2003
   (Religion or Belief) 2003
   (Sex Discrimination) 2005
   (Age) 2006

These laws forbid discrimination in employment or in providing education or training. They cover discrimination on the grounds of gender, race, disability, sexual orientation and religion or belief.

Disability

Disability Discrimination Act 1995

This Act was passed to end the discrimination that many disabled people face. It protects disabled people in employment, access to goods, facilities and services.

Mental Health

Mental Health Act 2007

This deals with people who have a mental illness with a view to their own safety and that of the general public.

Children

The Convention on the Rights of the Child 1989

Gives people under 18 extra protection not needed by adults.

Children Act 2004

By integrating services this Act aims to ensure that every child has the support that they need to:
- be healthy;
- stay safe;
- enjoy and achieve;
- make a positive contribution;
- achieve economic well-being.

Care

Nursing and Residential Care Homes Regulations 1984 (amended 2002)

These regulations require the regulation and inspection of nursing homes, residential homes for adults, children's homes, residential family centres and boarding schools.

Care Standards Act 2000

This Act required Social Care Councils to be set up to regulate the social care profession. Their functions include:
- enforcing standards of conduct and practice within the social care workforce,
- registering social care workers and regulating their conduct and training;
- ensuring that service users, carers, practitioners, employers and the general public have confidence the standards that are set for social care.

> **The four Social Care Councils in the UK**
>
> The General Social Care Council (for England)
>
> The Care Council of Wales
>
> The Scottish Social Services Council
>
> The Northern Ireland Social Care Council

Activity

Using the internet, obtain a copy of the information on the home page of each of the four Social Care Councils. Compare them, then note ways in which they are similar and ways in which they differ.

1. a Name three sets of laws and rules that protect the rights of individuals.

b Sixteen laws are mentioned on pages 84–85. Starting with the earliest law (1950), name each and give its purpose. Place your answer in a table.

Codes of practice and charters

Codes of practice

Codes of practice provide a clear guide for all those who work in health and social care. They set out the standards of practice and conduct that workers and their employers should meet. The aim is to improve levels of professionalism and public protection. Social care workers and nurses who break the codes may be removed from the social care and nursing registers. Codes of Practice for Social Care Workers and their employers are discussed on page 19.

Organisational policies and procedures

Policies are statements made by organisations to determine how codes of practice and statutory requirements are implemented in an organisation. An example is an organisation's equal opportunities policy.

Charters

A charter is a document that sets out the service that users can expect to receive. Charters are used by health authorities to publicise the available services and to improve the quality of them. For example, the Patient's Charter for England lays down patients' rights and the standards that patients can expect to be met.

Activity

Choose a health or social care setting, then select one piece of legislation and one code of practice that aims to support the rights of the individuals in that setting. Then:

i   **describe** the chosen legislation and code of practice;

ii **explain** how they can support the rights of the individuals in that setting;

iii **evaluate** (give your opinion) on how effective the legislation is in valuing diversity, promoting equality and supporting the rights of individuals in health and social care environments.

Chapter 5
How the body works

This chapter covers:

- The organisation of the cells, tissues, organs and systems in the human body.

- The structure, function and inter-relationships of the major systems in the body.

- Monitoring body systems through routine measurements and observations.

- Malfunctions of the body systems and the resultant needs of patients and service users.

The human body

In order to understand the principles of health and well-being, it is necessary to know about the structure of the body and its various parts (**anatomy**), how the body works (**physiology**) and the study of the mind (**psychology**).

The body consists of billions of individual cells organised into tissues, organs and systems:

- a **cell** is a tiny unit of living matter; there are many types of cells, for example red blood cells, muscle cells and nerve cells;
- a **tissue** is a group of cells specialised to perform a particular function, for example muscle tissue and brain tissue;
- an **organ** is a part of the body with a special function or functions, for example heart, skin, stomach;
- a **system** is a group of organs working together to carry out one or more functions, for example respiratory system, blood system.

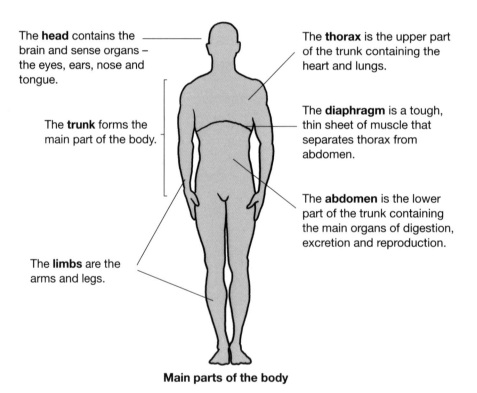

The **head** contains the brain and sense organs – the eyes, ears, nose and tongue.

The **trunk** forms the main part of the body.

The **limbs** are the arms and legs.

The **thorax** is the upper part of the trunk containing the heart and lungs.

The **diaphragm** is a tough, thin sheet of muscle that separates thorax from abdomen.

The **abdomen** is the lower part of the trunk containing the main organs of digestion, excretion and reproduction.

Main parts of the body

1. **a** Explain the meaning of the terms anatomy, physiology and psychology.
   b What does the human body consist of?
   c Explain the difference between cells, tissues, organs and systems.
   d i What occupies about half the head?
   ii Name the sense organs in the head.
   e i Name the two parts of the trunk,
   ii what separates them?
   f What are limbs?

Activity

Examine a model of the human body that shows the shape and size of the organs and how they fit together.

Inside the body

skin:
• covers and protects the body;
• is sensitive to touch, pain and the temperature outside the body;
• helps control the temperature inside the body.

heart – pumps blood around the body.

liver – the largest gland in the body with many functions including:
• produces bile to digest fat;
• removes alcohol, drugs and other unwanted substances from blood for elimination from the body;
• helps to keep the body warm from the heat it produces.

kidneys – remove waste substances and unwanted water from the blood to make urine.

bladder – stores urine.

brain:
• receives information from the sense organs;
• controls muscle movements;
• controls intelligence, emotions, personality and knowing who we are.

lungs – the place where the body takes in oxygen and expels carbon dioxide.

stomach – stores and digests food.

pancreas – produces:
• pancreatic juice that helps to digest food;
• hormones that control blood sugar.

intestines:
• continue the digestion of food;
• absorb water and particles of digested food into the blood stream.

Organs in the human body and their main function

Front of body

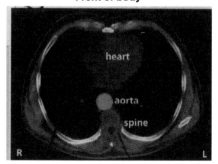

Thorax seen from below

Front of body

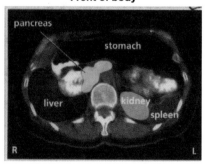

Abdomen seen from below

Activities

1. Draw a diagram of the human body to show the main organs. Label the organs and give at least one function of each.
2. Use the scans to draw and label a diagram of a section through the thorax and the abdomen.

2. **a** Name the organs in the thorax.
   b Give the function of the heart.
   c On its journey round the body, where does blood:
      i collect oxygen,
      ii obtain food,
      iii get rid of carbon dioxide,
      iv get rid of other waste substances?
   d Where is urine:
      i made,
      ii stored?
   e Name four organs concerned with the digestion of food.
   f Which organ:
      i produces heat,
      ii helps control body temperature,
      iii controls muscle movements?

Systems

Nine body systems are shown below and, by working together, they enable the body to function as a whole. Being inter-related, the malfunctioning of one system can affect the health of the whole body.

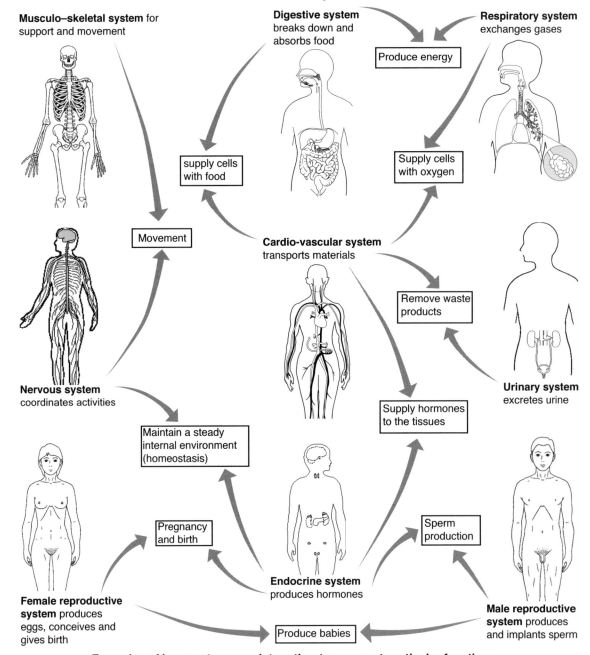

Musculo–skeletal system for support and movement

Digestive system breaks down and absorbs food

Respiratory system exchanges gases

Produce energy

supply cells with food

Supply cells with oxygen

Movement

Cardio-vascular system transports materials

Remove waste products

Nervous system coordinates activities

Urinary system excretes urine

Maintain a steady internal environment (homeostasis)

Supply hormones to the tissues

Pregnancy and birth

Sperm production

Female reproductive system produces eggs, conceives and gives birth

Endocrine system produces hormones

Produce babies

Male reproductive system produces and implants sperm

Examples of how systems work together to carry out particular functions

3. **a** Name the nine systems above and give the function of each.
   b Complete a table of the ten examples shown above of systems working together for a particular function.

Two systems working together	The function they carry out
Digestive and cardio-vascular systems	

The skin

The skin is the outer covering that **protects** the body from damage and disease, **controls** the amount of water lost through the skin, helps to **regulate** body temperature, **produces** vitamin D and melanin, and is **sensitive** to touch, temperature and pain. There are two main layers of skin:

- the **epidermis** is the outer layer of skin. The innermost cells continuously produce the new cells. These push the older cells up to the surface where they die through lack of food and oxygen. The dead cells then form a tough outer layer that protects the delicate tissues underneath.
- the **dermis** is the inner layer of skin. It contains blood vessels, nerves, hair roots and sweat glands held together by connective tissue. Wrinkles develop when this tissue loses its elasticity due to the natural process of ageing.

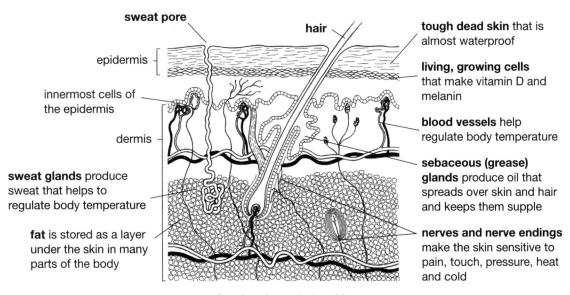

Section through the skin

Skin and hair colour

Cells in the innermost part of the epidermis produce melanin, which gives colour to hair and skin. In pale-skinned people, skin colour is also affected by the amount of blood in the skin making it look flushed (red) when the body is hot, and pale or slightly blue when the body is cold.

1. a List five functions of the skin.
  b Name the two main layers of the skin.
  c How do new cells in the epidermis become flakes of dead skin?
  d What is produced by sweat glands and sebaceous glands?
  e What makes the skin almost waterproof?
  f Name two parts that help regulate body temperature.
  g What makes the skin sensitive?
  h Where is fat stored?
  i What gives hair its colour?
  j Give two sources of skin colour in pale-skinned people.
  k Why do wrinkles develop?

Activity

a Draw a simple diagram of the skin. Then colour:
- nerve and nerve endings – dark blue;
- living cells of epidermis – pink, blood vessels – red;
- sebaceous glands – pale green, sweat gland – blue;
- hair – your own hair colour, fat layer – yellow;
- dead skin – no colour.

b Label and give the function of each part.
c Explain how the structure of the skin enables it to carry out its function.

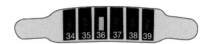

Forehead strip thermometer is the easiest to use and does not need batteries, but the readings are not so accurate as the other thermometers.

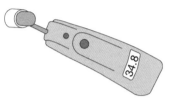

Forehead digital thermometer for placing against the skin.

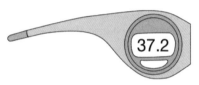

Mouth thermometer for placing under the tongue.

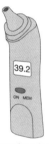

Ear thermometer for placing in the ear.

Different types of thermometer

Body temperature

Body temperature is the temperature of the inside of the body. The heat that keeps the body warm is produced mainly by the liver and the muscles, and it is lost mainly through the skin. When feeling cold, the normal response is to put on more clothes, to take some exercise or move to a warmer place. Opposite actions are taken when feeling hot.

Normal body temperature

The body temperature of healthy adults stays more or less constant within the range of 36.0 and 37.4°C. It is usually a little lower in the morning and a little higher in the late afternoon. There are slight differences when the temperature is measured on the forehead or in the mouth, armpit, ear or rectum. (➲ page 135 'Regulation of body temperature'.)

Fever is a rise in body temperature above normal. It is usually caused by bacterial or viral infection. A rise above 40.5°C may cause **delirium** (mental confusion), and young children may also suffer **convulsions** (unnatural jerking movements).

A person with a high fever can be cooled down by sponging with tepid water. Heat will then be lost from the body as the water evaporates.

Hypothermia

Hypothermia is a condition in which normal body temperature drops below 35°C (95°F). Those most at risk are:

- **older people**. The ability to regulate body temperature is reduced in old age. Therefore elderly people may not be aware of feeling cold even when their body temperature is very low. Also, those who have mobility problems may not generate much heat energy, or they may not eat enough, or their rooms may be too cold due to lack of heating.
- **babies**. The ability to regulate body temperature is not fully developed in babies, and they quickly lose body heat, unless dressed warmly, if they stay in a cold place for too long.

Activity

Using at least two different types of thermometer, take the temperature on your forehead, in your mouth and under your arm. Write up your results and conclusions. Compare your results with those of other students.

2. **a** What is body temperature?
   b Describe the normal body temperature of a healthy adult.
   c What is fever, and the usual cause?
   d What is meant by delirium and convulsions?
   e **i** What is hypothermia?
      ii Describe two groups of people who are most at risk from this condition, and explain why.
   f Describe four types of thermometer and say whether each is indicating a high, normal or low body temperature.

Skin disorders

Disorders of the skin may cause pain, itching and damage. If they affect a person's appearance, they can also cause distress and loss of self-esteem.

Rash is an outbreak of red spots or patches on the skin. It is usually due to an infectious disease or an allergy. **Allergy** is an adverse (bad) reaction to a particular substance that gets into the body, for example certain foods and bee or wasp stings.

Cold sores occur around the nose and mouth. They are caused by a virus and usually respond well to special cream obtainable from pharmacies.

Acne is a skin disorder common in adolescence. It is due to the over-activity and infection of the sebaceous glands. 'Spots' appear ranging from blackheads to painful red nodules.

Eczema is when parts of the skin become dry, red and very itchy. Scratching can lead to damage and infection. Eczema can be caused by an allergy.

An **ulcer** is a break in any surface inside or outside the body that fails to heal. For example, stomach ulcers, bedsores, genital ulcers and ulcers on the legs.

Activities

1. Explain the link between bedsores and the care that the patient receives.
2. Explain how the skin and blood system interrelate to keep the body temperature constant. (➲ page 135.)

Care of the skin

Washing

People who are clean feel more comfortable and are more pleasant to be with than people who are not. Being more hygienic, they are less prone to infection. A regular routine for washing and bathing is therefore an essential part of caring for patients and clients. Points to note are:

- use warm water and soap for washing;
- dry by patting gently with a clean towel as rubbing briskly may damage tender skin;
- use moisturising cream to soften dry, sore skin;
- use lip salve or Vaseline® for cracked lips.

Pressure sores

Pressure sores are ulcerated patches of the skin on the buttocks, heels or elbows of patients confined to bed. They occur in places where the constant pressure of the weight of the body stops blood from reaching those areas. The first warning sign is redness of the area and, unless the pressure is relieved, ulcers rapidly develop. Pressure sores are almost entirely prevented by good nursing. The patient's position should be changed frequently to allow blood to flow to the areas at risk, and the skin kept clean and dry.

3. a Give five possible effects of skin disorders.
   b Describe a skin disorder that:
      i   is common in adolescence,
      ii fails to heal,
      iii occurs around the mouth,
      iv is an outbreak of red spots,
      v   is very itchy.
   c When caring for patients:
      i   why is washing important?
      ii give four points to note.
   d i   What are bedsores,
      ii where do they occur,
      iii how can good nursing prevent them?

Musculo-skeletal system

The **musculo-skeletal system** consists of bones, joints and the muscles connected with them. Its functions are:

- **support** – the skeleton supports the body;
- **movement** – the muscles enable the body to move.

Skeleton

The skeleton is a rigid framework of bones that gives shape to the body, protects and supports the internal organs, provides attachment for muscles and ligaments, and enables movement.

skull { cranium / mandible
clavicle
scapula
sternum
humerus
radius
ulna
carpals
metacarpals
femur
patella
tibia
fibula
tarsals
metatarsals

skull protects the brain, ears, eyes and mouth.

rib cage protects the heart and lungs, and assists with breathing.

backbone (spine; vertebral column) encloses and protects the spinal cord, and supports the top half of the body.

discs of cartilage separate the small bones of the backbone; they act as shock-absorbers and allow the backbone to bend and turn.

pelvis supports and protects the organs in the lower abdomen.

arms, legs and **backbone** consist of a number of bones that fit closely together at the joints. **Joints** in the skeleton allow the body to move in different ways and carry out different types of movement; for example, the back can bend and turn, and the fingers can use a keyboard.

Activity inside bones

Bones are living structures and this is why they can grow during childhood and mend if they are broken. Blood vessels penetrate throughout bone tissue to provide materials to keep it alive. Red blood cells and some of the white cells are made in the marrow found inside many bones.

Osteoporosis

Osteoporosis is loss of bone tissue but not bone shape, making bones weaker and more liable to fracture. This condition is common in older people, especially women. Exercise and calcium and vitamin D in the diet may help to prevent the condition or delay its **onset** (beginning).

1. a i Describe two functions of the musculo-skeletal system.
  ii Give four functions of the skeleton.
b Give the anatomical name for:
  i jawbone,
  ii collar bone,
  iii shoulder blade,
  iv breast bone,
  v hip bone,
  vi bone in the upper arm,
  vii bones in the forearm,
  viii thigh bone,
  ix bones in the lower leg,
  x wrist bones,
  xi ankle bones.
c Which bones protect the:
  i brain,
  ii heart and lungs,
  iii spinal cord?
d Why can broken bones mend?
e What is made in bone marrow?
f i What is osteoporosis,
  ii who is most likely to suffer from the condition,
  iii what may help to delay onset?

Activity

a Label the bones in a diagram of the skeleton.
b Describe the skeleton, and how different parts of the skeleton relate to its functions.

Joints

The place where two bones meet is called a **joint**. Movement takes place at joints called synovial joints, for example, elbow, hip, jaw and at the places where the ribs connect with the backbone. Bones can move easily against each other because of the layer of smooth cartilage that covers the ends of the bones and the presence of fluid which lubricates ('oils') it.

Arthritis

Arthritis is inflammation at a joint. Inflamed joints are painful, swollen and stiff. Treatment is usually with pain relievers and anti-inflammatory drugs to reduce the swelling. It is possible to replace some badly affected joints with artificial ones.

Osteo-arthritis ('wear and tear') arthritis mostly affects the weight-bearing joints of the hips and knees. The cartilage covering the bones at the joints becomes damaged and movement becomes difficult and painful. Osteo-arthritis chiefly occurs in the elderly and those who are overweight. It may also develop in much-used thumb joints and in the joints of athletes.

Rheumatoid arthritis affects mainly the small joints in the fingers and toes. The disease can start suddenly in an otherwise fit person, and in women more often than men. The condition follows an 'up and down' course over weeks and months. Some people recover completely; others have permanently changed joints such as gnarled hands after the swelling has gone.

Ligaments

Ligaments are bands of tough tissue linking bones at a joint. They can bend but not stretch and so limit the range that a joint can move. If movement is pushed too far, the ligament will tear and the joint may be **dislocated** – a bone pushed out of its normal position. A **sprain** is a partly torn ligament, mostly occurring in ankles and knees, and needs time to heal.

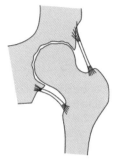

Diagram of a hip joint damaged by osteoarthritis

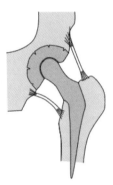

Diagram of a hip joint replacement

Activities

1. Draw and label diagrams to show **i** a hip joint damaged by osteoarthritis, **ii** a hip-joint replacement.
2. Search the internet for information about the care and treatment that could be given to patients with the two types of arthritis. Summarise the information from at least two documents, each document being at least 500 words long.
   (➲ Media search page 245.)

Comparing osteoarthritis with rheumatoid arthritis		
	Osteoarthritis	**Rheumatoid arthritis**
Which parts of the body are affected? What age group is mainly affected? What are the symptoms? Do people recover from the condition?		

2. **a** What is a joint?
   b When can bones at a joint move easily?
   c i What is arthritis?
   ii How does arthritis affect joints?
   iii What is the usual treatment?
   d What is a sprain, and what is a ligament?
   e When is a shoulder dislocated?
   f Copy and complete the table above.

Muscles

Muscle is the most abundant tissue in the body and it carries out all the body's movements. For example, the muscles attached to the skeleton move the bones, the heart muscle moves blood around the body, and the activity of muscles in the walls of the stomach and intestines moves food through the digestive system.

Skeletal muscles

These muscles are attached to bones either directly or by tendons. A **tendon** is a tough, white cord that attaches a muscle to a bone. Movement of muscles is under the control of the nervous system. If we want to run, sit or chew, messages from the brain are sent along nerves to the appropriate muscles to move the right bones. Muscles need to be used to keep them in good condition because, when not used, they waste away. A certain amount of exercise is therefore essential to keep the muscles in good working order.

Activities

1. Describe the function of muscle tissue.
2. Describe skeletal muscles.
3. Use labelled diagrams to explain the structure of skeletal muscles in relation to their functions.

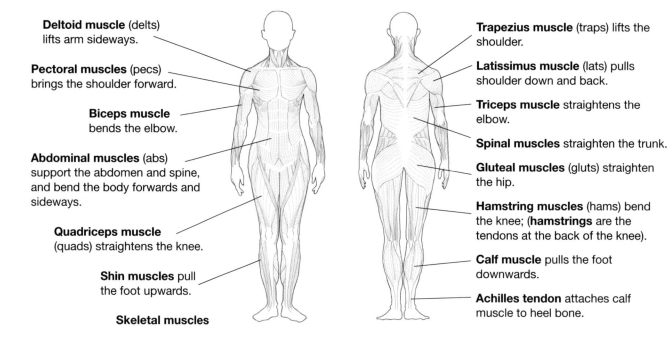

Deltoid muscle (delts) lifts arm sideways.

Pectoral muscles (pecs) brings the shoulder forward.

Biceps muscle bends the elbow.

Abdominal muscles (abs) support the abdomen and spine, and bend the body forwards and sideways.

Quadriceps muscle (quads) straightens the knee.

Shin muscles pull the foot upwards.

Skeletal muscles

Trapezius muscle (traps) lifts the shoulder.

Latissimus muscle (lats) pulls shoulder down and back.

Triceps muscle straightens the elbow.

Spinal muscles straighten the trunk.

Gluteal muscles (gluts) straighten the hip.

Hamstring muscles (hams) bend the knee; (**hamstrings** are the tendons at the back of the knee).

Calf muscle pulls the foot downwards.

Achilles tendon attaches calf muscle to heel bone.

3. a i Which is the most abundant tissue in the body, ii what is its function? iii Give three examples.
   b i How are muscles attached to the bones, ii what is a tendon?
     iii Name the tendons shown above (two answers).
   c i How are skeletal muscles controlled? ii Give one example.
   d i Why do muscles need to be used, ii what keeps them in good condition?
   e What are tendons?

f Skeletal muscles		
Common name (if there is one)	**Anatomical name** (if given)	**Action**
Delts	Deltoid muscle	

Muscular and related disorders

Muscular dystrophy

Muscular dystrophy is a rare inherited disorder in which muscles are weak and waste away. A common form is **Duchenne's muscular dystrophy** that only occurs in boys. The disease cannot be cured, but physiotherapy and support equipment such as calliper splints can help in living with the condition.

Dyspraxia

Dyspraxia is extreme clumsiness due to the poor coordination of muscle movements by the brain. The condition does not affect a child's intelligence but it does reduce the ability to learn physical skills.

Tendonitis

This is inflammation of a tendon. It is commonly caused by overuse or injury to a particular tendon, especially those of the shoulder, elbow, wrist, finger, thigh, knee or back of the heel (Achilles tendon). Symptoms include pain when the affected tendons are being used.

Repetitive strain injury (RSI)

RSI is an umbrella term referring to injuries to muscles, tendons and nerves caused by repetitive movements usually of the hands, wrists or shoulders.

Symptoms include:
- inflammation of the tendons and joints of the hands and arms;
- tenderness or pain in the muscles and joints;
- tingling ('pins and needles') or numbness in the hand or arm;
- loss of strength or sensation in the hand.

RSI is linked to repetitive work, for example using a computer or vibrating equipment. When symptoms occur, it is important to get early advice to prevent long-term damage.

CFS/ME

Chronic fatigue syndrome (CFS) is also known as **myalgic encephalomyelitis** (ME). The main symptom is persistent tiredness and exhaustion that does not go away with sleep or rest. Other symptoms can include muscle and joint pains, headaches and poor concentration. It tends to last for months or years, but most people eventually recover.

Activity

Choose a muscular or related disorder, then:
i describe the disorder in not less than 500 words,
ii find some statistics relating to the disorder.

---

4. a i What is muscular dystrophy,
     ii which is a common form,
     iii what help can be given?
   b What is dyspraxia?
   c i What is tendonitis,
     ii where is it most likely to occur,
     iii what is a symptom?
   d i What is RSI,
     ii what is it linked with,
     iii what are some symptoms,
     iv why is urgent treatment important?
   e i What is CFS/ME,
     ii what is the main symptom,
     iii what are other symptoms,
     iv how long does the disorder last?

Physiotherapy

Physiotherapy is treatment that helps the body to recover after injury or illness. It aims to improve patients' mobility and quality of life. It is used for example to:

- help recovery after accidents such as broken legs and head injuries;
- rehabilitate patients following a stroke;
- improve the quality of life of children with cerebral palsy;
- help patients to expand and clear their lungs after operations;
- help recovery from back and neck pain, torn muscles and ligaments, and sports injuries.

A range of techniques is used such as manipulation, exercise, electrotherapy, hydrotherapy and acupuncture.

Manipulation

Manipulation is the skilled use of the hands to restore movement to patients' stiff and painful joints. It is often applied on the back and neck, and also to other joints such as shoulders, elbows and knees. It helps to relieve tension in the muscles, which allows the joints to move freely again, and it is useful for people of all ages.

Exercises

Exercises are designed to strengthen and lengthen muscles and improve the range of movement of the joints. The physiotherapist advises patients on which exercises to do for their condition, and shows them how to do them safely. Exercises of the right type can, for example:

- strengthen muscles and joints and increase the range of movement after ligament tears, fractured bones or joint replacement surgery;
- enable patients to walk normally after having a leg in a plaster cast following a **fracture** (broken bone) in the leg;
- help stroke victims recover the use of affected muscles;
- enable asthmatics to breathe more efficiently;
- help recovery from back pain and sciatica and prevent recurrence.

5. **a** What is physiotherapy and what are its aims?
   b Why may physiotherapy be given:
   i after an accident,
   ii to stroke patients,
   iii to children with cerebral palsy,
   iv following an operation,
   v for sports injuries?
   c Name five techniques used by physiotherapists.
   d i What is manipulation,
   ii when is it applied,
   iii what is its effect?
   e What is the purpose of exercises?
   f In what way can exercise help patients:
   i after joint replacement surgery,
   ii who have had a leg in plaster,
   iii with asthma,
   iv who have had a stroke,
   v with sciatica?

Activity

Explain how the skeleton and muscles inter-relate to allow the body to move.

Electro-therapy

The most commonly-used forms of electro-therapy are ultrasound and TENS.

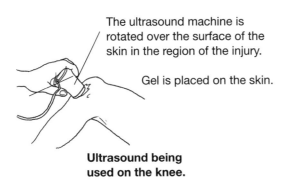

The ultrasound machine is rotated over the surface of the skin in the region of the injury.

Gel is placed on the skin.

Ultrasound being used on the knee.

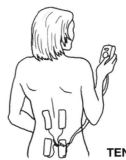

TENS machine being used to relieve back pain.

Ultrasound uses sound waves at frequencies higher than can be heard by the human ear to speed the rate of healing of tissues beneath the surface of the skin. It is used to speed up the repair of recently injured muscles and ligaments.

TENS (Transcutaneous Electrical Nerve Stimulation) is used to reduce pain. It produces a tingling sensation in the skin that helps to mask the pain and allows early movement of injured muscles and joints. This encourages better healing of the tissues and their return to normal function. TENS is also used to ease the pain of childbirth.

Acupuncture

Acupuncture is a form of pain relief invented by the Chinese more than two thousand years ago. It uses very fine needles which pass through the skin. Physiotherapists use acupuncture to relieve pain and this enables patients to exercise. Exercise helps muscles to return to normal movement and function.

Hydrotherapy

Hydrotherapy is physiotherapy exercises carried out in warm water. The water supports the body so that weak muscles and stiff joints can move more easily. This treatment is used, for example, to:

* restore function to a fractured limb that has been immobilised in a cast for several weeks;
* strengthen weak muscles following a stroke;
* loosen stiff muscles of children with cerebral palsy.

Flotation belt

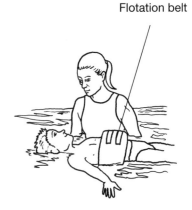

Activity

Invite a physiotherapist to talk about his/her work, or obtain a CD or DVD about the profession.
i   Produce a poster advertising the event.
ii Write a report about the talk/video in at least 500 words.
    (➲ Writing a report, page 242.)

6. a Name two forms of electrotherapy.
  b i What does ultrasound use,
    ii when is it used?
  c Describe how TENS helps the healing process.
  d What is the purpose of acupuncture?
  e i What is hydrotherapy,
    ii what is the effect of water on the body,
    iii when may this treatment be used?

Cardio-vascular system

The **cardio-vascular system** includes the heart and the network of blood vessels. Its function is to transport blood around the body.

Blood

Blood flows around the body in the blood vessels. Its function is to transport substances from one part of the body to another. For example blood carries:

- oxygen from the lungs to the tissues;
- carbon dioxide from the tissues to the lungs;
- food from the digestive system to the tissues;
- waste products from the tissues to the kidneys and liver;
- hormones from the various glands where they are made to the parts of the body that they affect;
- white cells and antibodies to protect against infection;
- heat produced by the liver and muscles to all parts of the body.

Activity

Describe how the structure of blood enables it to carry out its function.

1. a Describe the cardio-vascular system.
b i Give the function of blood.
ii What is blood a mixture of?
c When plasma is analysed:
i which is the main substance?
ii name other substances present,
iii what other substances may be found?
d i Are there more red or white cells,
ii why does the body need both red and white cells?
e Explain the colour change of blood from bright red to almost black.
f i What is a bruise?
ii How can you tell a fresh bruise from an older bruise?
g When do blood clots form?
h When are blood clots:
i useful,
ii dangerous?

Plasma is a pale yellow fluid containing many substances including:
- water – 90% of plasma is water;
- carbon dioxide;
- glucose (blood sugar);
- antibodies – protect against various diseases;
- hormones, e.g. thyroid hormone;
- vitamins, e.g. vitamin D, vitamin B_{12}
- minerals, e.g. iron and calcium.
It may also contain:
- nicotine from smoke;
- alcohol (important in drink-driving cases);
- medicines;
- illegal drugs.

White cells help to protect the body against infection by destroying germs or producing antibodies against them.

Red cells carry oxygen to all parts of the body. Red cells only last for about 120 days and are constantly replaced.

When a blood sample is left to stand it separates into the three layers shown above

Colour Blood changes colour according to the amount of oxygen it contains. Blood containing oxygen is bright red. As it loses oxygen it turns to dark red, and when all the oxygen has gone it is very dark blue/black.

Bruise A **bruise** is bleeding under the skin. At first it is red or pink, then gradually becomes dark blue. It changes to greenish yellow as the blood is gradually broken down and removed.

Clotting A blood clot is a semi-solid mass of blood. It normally forms when the skin is damaged. This stops blood leaking from the body and also prevents germs from entering the wound. A blood clot can also form inside the body when blood vessels are damaged; this can result in a heart attack, stroke or deep vein thrombosis (DVT).

Blood tests

Blood tests are carried out for many reasons, including:

- **the function of an organ** can be checked such as the liver, thyroid, bone marrow or kidneys;
- **when a disease is suspected**, a blood test can confirm a diagnosis, for example:
- a low level of haemoglobin can indicate anaemia,
- increased numbers of white blood cells can indicate an infection or leukaemia,
- a high level of blood glucose can indicate diabetes,
- a high level of cholesterol can indicate an increased risk of heart attack and stroke,
- **the progress of an illness** can be monitored to find out how well the treatment is working;
- **a blood test for HIV** shows whether an individual is infected and, if so, can give an early warning before the disease develops;
- **before giving a blood transfusion** – this is essential to make sure that the blood of the patient and the blood being transfused are compatible for:
- blood group (A, B, AB or O),
- rhesus factor (Rh positive or Rh negative).

Blood disorders

Anaemia

Anaemia is a shortage of haemoglobin in the blood. The main symptoms are tiredness and breathlessness. **Haemoglobin** contains iron and is the red substance in red blood cells that carries oxygen. Anaemia develops due to:

- **haemorrhage** (rapid loss of blood) after an accident;
- **iron-deficiency** caused by a low-iron diet without meat, eggs or vegetables, increased need during puberty and pregnancy;
- **a slow rate of blood loss** due to heavy periods or to bleeding into the intestines from a stomach ulcer, cancer or ulcerative colitis.

Leukaemia

Leukaemia is caused by the over-production of abnormal white cells. There are several types of leukaemia and they are all forms of cancer, many of which respond well to treatment.

High cholesterol

Cholesterol is a fatty substance present in blood and is an essential part of a healthy body. The recommended level of blood cholesterol is under 5 mmol/litre. Levels above 6 are regarded as high and a risk factor for heart attacks and stroke.

2. a i Why is a patient's blood tested before a transfusion is given?
   ii Name three other reasons for a blood test.
 b i What is anaemia?
   ii What is haemoglobin?
   iii What are the symptoms of anaemia?
   iv When may anaemia develop?
 c i What is leukaemia?
   ii What blood test is carried out to check for leukaemia?
 d Why is blood tested for:
   i blood sugar,
   ii HIV,
   iii cholesterol?
 e i What is cholesterol,
   ii what is the recommended cholesterol level in blood?

Activity

Carry out a media search for one of the blood disorders on this page. Identify the risk factors and describe the care and treatment that can be given. (➲ Media search, page 245.)

Heart

The human heart is about the size of a fist. It is a pump that beats continuously throughout life to keep blood circulating around the body. The heart is made of muscle which, like all muscles, contracts and relaxes. The **heartbeat** is the result of the alternate contraction and relaxation of the heart muscle.

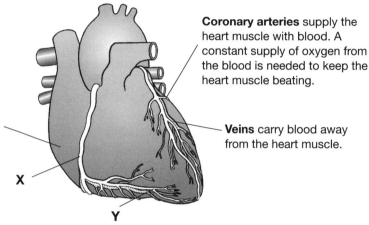

Coronary arteries supply the heart muscle with blood. A constant supply of oxygen from the blood is needed to keep the heart muscle beating.

Heart muscle (the wall of the heart).

Veins carry blood away from the heart muscle.

X

Y

The heart from the outside

Coronary heart disease

Coronary heart disease develops when the coronary arteries become partly or completely blocked either by a build up of fatty material (➲ page 106) or a blood clot. The result can be angina or a heart attack.

A **heart attack** is the death of a part of the heart muscle. It occurs when its blood supply is interrupted by a block in a coronary artery. This causes pain in the centre of the chest, which often spreads to the neck and arms. Whether a heart attack is mild or severe depends on where the blockage takes place, and how much of the heart muscle is damaged. On the diagram above:

* if a blockage occurs at Y, only a small part of the heart muscle is affected and the heart usually continues to beat normally;
* if a blockage occurs at X, much more muscle is damaged and the heartbeat may be weaker.

Angina refers to pain in the centre of the chest. It happens because the coronary arteries have become partly blocked ('furred up') and are unable to supply enough oxygenated blood to the heart muscle when it is working hard. Angina occurs when increased demands are made on the heart by exercise, cold weather, digestion or excitement. It disappears with relaxation and warmth.

Activity

Draw a diagram of the heart and shade in the areas that would be affected by a blood clot at X and at Y. Use your diagram to explain the difference between a mild and a severe heart attack.

3. **a i** What is the function of the heart,
   ii what is the heart wall made of,
   iii what is the heartbeat?
   b When does coronary heart disease develop, and what can it result in?
   c i What is angina,
   ii why does it occur,
   iii when does it occur,
   iv what relieves it?
   d i What is a heart attack,
   ii where is pain felt,
   iii why may it be mild or severe?

Inside the heart

The heart is composed of four chambers - right atrium, right ventricle, left atrium and left ventricle. Although the right and left sides of the heart are joined together, the blood in them is completely separate and does not mix. The left ventricle has a thicker wall than the right ventricle because it needs more muscle power to pump blood to all parts of the body. The right ventricle pumps blood only to the lungs.

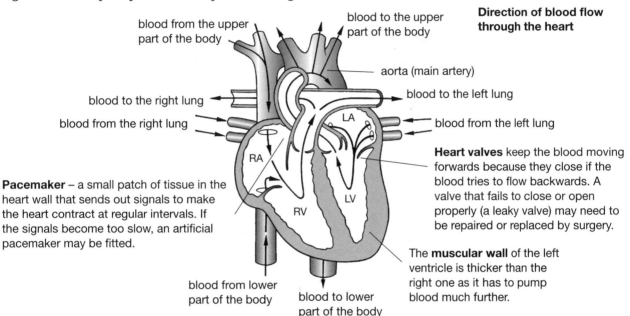

Direction of blood flow through the heart

blood from the upper part of the body

blood to the upper part of the body

aorta (main artery)

blood to the right lung

blood from the right lung

blood to the left lung

blood from the left lung

LA

RA

RV

LV

Pacemaker – a small patch of tissue in the heart wall that sends out signals to make the heart contract at regular intervals. If the signals become too slow, an artificial pacemaker may be fitted.

Heart valves keep the blood moving forwards because they close if the blood tries to flow backwards. A valve that fails to close or open properly (a leaky valve) may need to be repaired or replaced by surgery.

The **muscular wall** of the left ventricle is thicker than the right one as it has to pump blood much further.

blood from lower part of the body

blood to lower part of the body

Heart failure

Heart failure is a misleading term. It means that the heart is not pumping as strongly as it should, not that it has failed to work altogether. Heart failure can be due to a number of causes, some of which can be corrected.

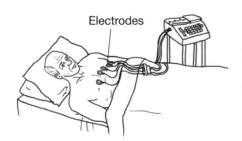

Electrodes

Electrocardiogram (ECG)
An ECG is a recording of the electrical activity of the heart. ECGs help in the diagnosis or monitoring of heart disease.

Activity

Draw a simple outline of the heart and:
i   name the four chambers,
ii colour in red – the blood in the left atrium and ventricle, and the blood vessels attached to them (red = oxygenated blood),
iii colour in blue – the blood in the right atrium and ventricle, and the blood vessels attached to them (blue = blood short of oxygen).

4. a i Give the initials and full names of the four chambers of the heart.
   ii Which chamber has the thickest wall?
   b Name the main artery from the heart.
   c i Where is the heart's pacemaker situated,
     ii what is its function,
     iii when may an artificial pacemaker be needed?
   d i What is the function of the heart valves,
     ii what is a leaky valve?
   e Why is 'heart failure' a misleading term?
   f i What does ECG stand for,
     ii what is its function,
     iii where are the electrodes placed?

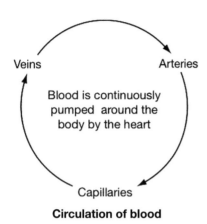

Circulation of blood

Blood vessels

Blood vessels are tubes through which blood flows as it circulates around the body. There are three different types:

- **arteries carry blood away from the heart**. The arteries give off branches to the various parts of the body. These in turn divide into smaller and smaller branches and, finally, into tiny capillaries that penetrate throughout all the tissues in the body.
- **capillaries link arteries to veins**. They have very thin walls and, as the blood flows through them, substances such as oxygen and food pass through the walls to the surrounding tissues, and waste materials such as carbon dioxide pass from the tissues to the blood.
- **veins return blood back to the heart**. Blood from the capillaries flows into small veins, and these link up to form larger and larger veins that eventually join the heart.

5. **a** What are blood vessels?
   b Name the three types of blood vessel.
   c i Is the larger blood vessel an artery or vein,
   ii what happens if it is cut,
   iii what is the colour of its blood and why?
   d How do the walls of arteries and veins differ?
   e i What is the function of the capillaries,
   ii what substances pass through their walls?
   f Describe how blood carried away from the heart in arteries is eventually returned back to the heart via the capillaries and veins.

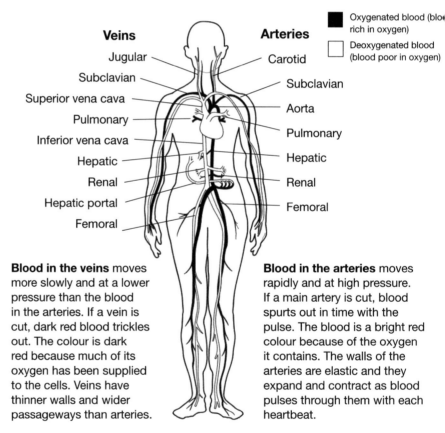

Blood in the veins moves more slowly and at a lower pressure than the blood in the arteries. If a vein is cut, dark red blood trickles out. The colour is dark red because much of its oxygen has been supplied to the cells. Veins have thinner walls and wider passageways than arteries.

Blood in the arteries moves rapidly and at high pressure. If a main artery is cut, blood spurts out in time with the pulse. The blood is a bright red colour because of the oxygen it contains. The walls of the arteries are elastic and they expand and contract as blood pulses through them with each heartbeat.

Main blood vessels

Activity

On a diagram of the main blood vessels:
i Colour in red all the blood vessels containing oxygenated blood, that is, all the arteries except the pulmonary artery, but including the pulmonary vein.
ii Colour in blue all the blood vessels containing blood that is short of oxygen, that is, all the veins except the pulmonary vein, but including the pulmonary artery.

Circulation

Blood continuously circulates from the heart to the lungs to collect oxygen, then back to the heart to be pumped to all the parts of the body before returning to the heart again. It takes about half a minute to complete the double circuit.

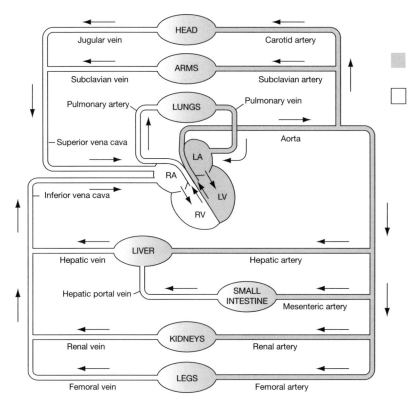

General plan of circulation

▨ Oxygenated blood
(blood rich in oxygen)

☐ Deoxygenated blood
(blood poor in oxygen)
A = atrium
L = left
R = right
V = ventricle

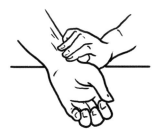

Taking the pulse at the wrist
(N.B. Don't use your thumb to take a pulse).

Pulse

The **pulse** is a wave of blood that is pumped through the arteries with each heartbeat. It can be felt in places where main arteries come close to the skin surface in the wrist and neck. In an adult, the pulse rate is 60-80 times a minute when resting. Exercise causes the pulse rate to increase and, during strenuous exercise, the rate can increase up to 200 beats per minute. The pulse is also increased by excitement, fear and some illnesses. An abnormally fast pulse when a person is resting can be a sign of infection.

6. **a** Calculate how many times blood circulates around the body in one day.
   b i What is the pulse,
   ii what is the pulse rate of a resting adult?
   iii Give four reasons for the pulse rate to increase.
   c Draw a diagram to show how to take the pulse in the wrist.
   d List the blood vessels and areas of the heart that blood passes through as it circulates from:
   i left atrium to kidneys (3 parts), **ii** arms to lungs (5 parts),
   iii liver to small intestine (11 parts), **iv** head to legs (11 parts).

Activity

This exercise requires two people **A** and **B**. **A** sits quietly for about ten minutes. **B** then takes **A**'s pulse for one minute and records the result. **A** takes vigorous exercise for a few minutes. **B** immediately takes **A**'s pulse for one minute, records the result, and continues to do this each minute until **A**'s pulse has returned to what it was before exercise was taken. Use the results to make a graph to show 'The effect of exercise on pulse rate'.

Disease of the arteries

Thickening of the arteries (atheroma)

The inner walls of arteries become thicker and less elastic when patches of fatty material called plaque form on them. As plaque builds up it reduces the space inside the arteries and can slow or stop the blood flow. This can result in:

- angina if narrowing occurs in a coronary artery;
- a heart attack, if a coronary artery is blocked;
- a stroke if an artery to the brain is blocked.

Plaque consists mainly of cholesterol and the build up of plaque in arteries is linked to a diet high in saturated fats, obesity, inactivity and smoking.

Activities

1. Using a computer, explain why a stroke occurs and describe the two main causes. Add additional information from the internet, for example:
   a the variety of symptoms shown by stroke victims;
   b a simple test to find out if someone may have had a stroke.
2. Describe the cardiovascular system, then explain how its structure relates to its function.

7. a i What is plaque,
   ii what does it consist of?
   b What is a build up of plaque in arteries linked with?
   c Name two conditions that can result from slow blood flow.
   d Use diagrams to show the difference between a healthy artery and a diseased artery.
   e What is a stroke?
   f Why is a continuous supply of oxygen essential for brain cells?
   g Describe the two main causes of stroke.

Inside a healthy artery

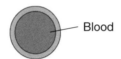

Blood

Blood can flow freely though a healthy artery. The artery wall expands with each heartbeat as a wave of blood is pumped through. This is felt as the pulse.

Inside a diseased artery

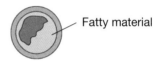

Fatty material

Fatty material deposited on the artery wall makes the wall thicker and less elastic and the space for blood to flow through is reduced.

Strokes

A **stroke** occurs when the normal blood supply to a part of the brain is cut off. Brain cells depend on a continuous supply of oxygen from the blood stream. When deprived of oxygen for more than about four minutes, brain cells can die and the functions controlled by that part of the brain cease resulting in, for example, paralysis (➲ page 121) down one side of the body.

There are two main causes of strokes:

- **a blood clot in an artery to the brain**. This restricts the amount of oxygen to the part of the brain supplied by that artery. If a small area is affected, only minor symptoms may occur. But if a large area is affected, it can cause severe symptoms, and even death.
- **bleeding into the brain**. If a weak artery bursts, blood escapes and damages neighbouring brain tissue. Other brain cells can also be damaged if their blood supply is reduced and they are not receiving enough oxygen.

Disease of the veins

DVT (Deep Vein Thrombosis)

A DVT is a blood clot in a vein, usually in the calf or thigh. It is more likely to occur when a person has been in the same position for a long time, and the blood in the vein moves so slowly that it clots. There is some discomfort, but the danger occurs if the clot becomes loose and travels in the blood stream through the heart to the lungs where it blocks the circulation in the lungs.

Varicose veins

Varicose veins are swollen veins usually seen on the legs. They occur when the valves in the veins become weak and fail to close properly, allowing blood to collect, causing the veins to swell and be painful. A tendency to varicose veins often runs in families. The condition can be caused by standing still for long periods, lack of exercise, being overweight or pregnant.

Blood pressure

Blood pressure (BP) is the pressure of blood in a main artery. It varies considerably between individuals, and also changes from minute to minute. Strenuous activity, anger or anxiety raise the blood pressure; rest and relaxation lower it. The BP of an adult when resting is typically about 120/80. The BP at rest tends to increase with increasing body weight.

High blood pressure (hypertension) is a blood pressure above the normal range expected when at rest (BP above 140/90). It rarely produces symptoms and a person may feel very well. But if the pressure is too high in the arteries, it can:

- damage tissues, for example in the kidneys and the eyes;
- break weaker arteries, causing strokes or heart attacks.

This is the reason for regular checks on blood pressure because, if it becomes raised, advice and treatment can be started before complications arise. Treatment is by medication and/or a change in lifestyle and needs to be checked regularly.

Low blood pressure When blood pressure is too low, not enough blood is supplied to the brain so, when standing, a person faints and falls to the ground. Recovery occurs rapidly when blood supplies reach the brain on lying down. BP low enough to cause symptoms is usually less than 90/60.

The pressure of blood pushes open the valve and allows the blood to flow through.

When the pressure is relaxed, the valve closes and stops blood flowing backwards.

Valves in the veins prevent blood flowing backwards.

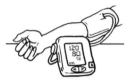

Measuring blood pressure
Two readings are taken that correspond with the rise and fall of pressure in an artery as a wave of blood moves through with each heartbeat. A result of '120/80' means that at every heartbeat, 120 is the highest pressure in the artery and 80 is the lowest.

Before high blood pressure is diagnosed it is usually measured on at least three different occasions. This is because some people become very anxious and need to get used to having their blood pressure taken.

8. **a** Why do veins have valves?
   b i What does DVT mean,
   ii why does it develop?
   c i What are varicose veins,
   ii why do they occur,
   iii when are they more likely to develop?
   d What is blood pressure?
   e Give the usual blood pressure of a young adult when resting.
   f What causes blood pressure to vary?
   g i What is hypertension,
   ii what are the symptoms,
   iii what damage can it do?
   h Why is blood pressure checked regularly?
   i How is blood pressure measured?
   j Why is one BP reading not a good basis for a diagnosis?
   k Describe the effects of low blood pressure.

Lymphatic system

The **lymphatic system** contains:

- **lymph nodes** (often called **glands**) which protect the body against infection by producing **lymphocytes** (one of the types of white blood cell) and **antibodies**;
- **Tonsils, spleen** and **thymus** also produce lymphocytes and antibodies and are important in building up the immune system in children;
- **lymph vessels** which remove fluid (**lymph**) from the tissues and prevent them from becoming waterlogged.

The **lymph vessels** form a network that penetrates to nearly all parts of the body. Fluid from the tissues drains into them and then flows back into the blood stream near the heart.

The **lymph nodes** are situated along the lymph vessels, and are found in clusters in the armpit, neck and groin. They:
- filter bacteria from the lymph as it flows through the lymph vessels;
- respond by producing more antibodies and lymphocytes when the body is infected by bacteria or viruses.

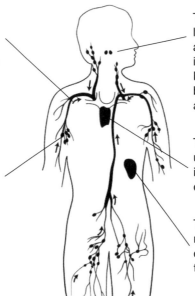

The **tonsils** are two almond-shaped lumps of lymph tissue one on each side at the back of the mouth. **Tonsillitis** is inflammation and infection of the tonsils. It is common in children but not adults because the tonsils almost disappear by adulthood.

The **thymus** is situated in the thorax underneath the top of the breastbone. It increases in size in childhood then almost disappears.

The **spleen** is situated in the abdomen near the stomach. It is very active in young children, helping them to develop immunity to disease.

Lymphatic system
→ pathway of the fluid (lymph) as it flows through the lymph vessels

Disorders of the lymphatic system

'Swollen glands' are enlarged lymph nodes. They swell when responding to infection. For example, the nodes swell in the neck in response to infection in the throat or scalp, and in the armpit in response to a septic finger. Some types of cancer can spread though lymph vessels and affect the lymph nodes they pass though.

Glandular fever is an infectious disease that affects the lymphatic system mainly in adolescents and young adults.

1. a What does the lymphatic system contain?
 b Describe two functions of the lymphatic system.
 c Describe the lymph vessels.
 d i Where are lymph nodes found,
  ii what are their functions?
 e i Where are the tonsils situated,
  ii what is tonsillitis,
  iii why is tonsillitis uncommon in adults?
 f i Where is the thymus situated,
  ii what happens to it?
 g i Where is the spleen situated,
  ii why is it more active in young children?
 h i What are swollen glands responding to?
  ii Give an example.
 i What is glandular fever?
 j How does fluid in the tissues reach the heart?

Immune system

The **immune system** uses lymphocytes to fight infections caused by germs. **Germs** are microbes (mainly bacteria and viruses) that cause disease. When germs get into the body, lymphocytes have two ways of fighting them:

- white blood cells that engulf (eat) the germs;
- antibodies are produced to destroy the germs.

Disease occurs when the germs multiply more quickly than they can be destroyed by antibodies and white blood cells.

How the immune system works

The immune system is able to recognise each type of germ and then make **antibodies** against them. Each type of germ results in its own type of antibody. Antibodies are made by lymphocytes in lymph nodes, bone marrow, thymus and spleen. They circulate in the blood stream and attack those germs that they 'recognise'.

Obtaining immunity

Antibodies to protect against infectious diseases are produced by:

- **natural immunity** – antibodies are produced when germs enter the body;
- **immunisation** (**vaccination**) – injection with a vaccine.

Types of vaccine

Active vaccine is made from a harmless form of a particular bacterium or virus. It stimulates the body to make antibodies against that germ without causing infection. This type of vaccine usually gives long-lasting protection against, for example, measles, mumps, rubella and TB.

Passive vaccines contain ready-made antibodies and are used to protect against rabies.

Auto-immune diseases

An auto-immune disease develops when the body produces antibodies that attack its own normal body cells. These diseases include a number of disorders such as rheumatoid arthritis and some cases of asthma.

Allergy

Allergy is an immune reaction by the body to a particular substance such as dust mites, pollen, pets and nuts.

Activity

Find out what vaccinations are available for:
i   children,
ii health and social care workers.
(➲ Media search page 245.)

2. a What causes infection?
   b Name two ways of fighting infection.
   c i   What are antibodies,
     ii where are they made,
     iii how do they act?
   d Describe two ways of obtaining immunity,
   e What are auto-immune diseases?
   f What is an allergy?

Respiratory system

The **respiratory system** is used for **breathing**, that is, the alternate **inhaling** (breathing in) and **exhaling** (breathing out) of air.

Nose warms inhaled air and filters out dust particles.

Throat (pharynx)

Tonsillitis is inflammation of the tonsils at the sides of the throat.

Rhinitis is inflammation of the lining of the nose due to allergy (e.g. hay fever) or infection (e.g. common cold). Excess mucus is produced and a blocked nose results.

Larynx (voice box)

Laryngitis is inflammation of the voice box.

Trachea (windpipe). The windpipe and the tubes in the lungs are kept open by cartilages in their walls.

Tracheitis is inflammation of the windpipe.

Bronchitis is infection of the air tubes by bacteria or viruses; bronchitis can either be acute (short-term) or chronic (long-term).

Pneumonia is inflammation of the lung tissue due to infection with bacteria or viruses.

Emphysema is the destruction of lung tissue.

Lung tissue consists of masses of air tubes and air sacs.

The **bronchi** divide and branch into smaller and smaller tubes (**bronchioles**) that reach all parts of the lung. Each tiny branch ends in an air sac.

Air sacs (alveoli) have very thin walls and expand when air is inhaled, then collapse when air is breathed out. They are surrounded by a network of capillaries (very tiny blood vessels ➲ page 106). The thin walls of both air sacs and capillaries allow gases (oxygen and carbon dioxide) to pass through them.

The respiratory system

Breathing continues throughout life in order to obtain oxygen and get rid of carbon dioxide. Oxygen is needed to release the energy locked up in food such as glucose. The carbon dioxide produced by this process must be removed to prevent it from poisoning the cells. With each breath:

- the lungs expand and air rushes in to fill up the space, passing through the nose or mouth, the windpipe, the tubes in the lungs and into the air sacs;
- oxygen from the air in the air sacs moves into the blood in the surrounding capillaries, and carbon dioxide moves in the opposite direction from blood to air;
- the lungs then contract and air is squeezed out of the lungs taking carbon dioxide with it.

Activities

1. a Draw and label a diagram of the respiratory system.
   b Explain how the structure of the respiratory system enables it to be used for breathing.
2. a Find out about a disease of the respiratory system.
   b Identify the risk factors associated with the disease.
   c Explain the care that needs to be given to patients with the disease (➲ Media search page 245).
3. Using text with images, produce an information leaflet for care workers that describes the disease.

1. a Give the function of the respiratory system.
   b i Why is breathing necessary for life,
      ii why is oxygen needed,
      iii what must be removed, and why?
   c Place these parts in the order that inhaled air passes through:
      air sacs bronchi trachea nose
      pharynx bronchioles larynx
   d i Draw a diagram of an air sac and surrounding blood vessels.
      ii What makes air sacs suitable for the exchange of gases?
      iii Which gas moves from air to blood, and which moves in the opposite direction?
   e Complete the chart for the seven diseases mentioned above.

Disease	Part of the body affected	Effect of disease
Rhinitis		

Breathing

It is possible to live for a couple of days without drinking water and a long time without food, but only a few minutes without breathing. Breathing is a regular and mainly automatic process. Air is alternately breathed into the lungs (inhaled) and then breathed out (exhaled). The way of breathing varies being:

- rapid and deep during exercise - to obtain extra oxygen and get rid of the extra carbon dioxide;
- rapid when angry;
- short and shallow when anxious;
- slow and regular when feeling calm and relaxed or asleep;
- hyperventilation (over-breathing) during a panic attack.

Hyperventilation is unnaturally fast, deep breathing that may occur at times of extreme anxiety or during a panic attack. It can be accompanied by dizziness or fainting, trembling, tingling and cramp in the hands. These symptoms are caused by loss of too much carbon dioxide from the blood.

Breathlessness is normal in healthy people when taking vigorous exercise. Breathlessness can also be caused by infections such as bronchitis and pneumonia.

Chronic (long-term) breathlessness is a sign of ill-health. Common causes are:

- smoking – lungs become clogged up with excess mucus (sputum), which encourages chronic bronchitis and emphysema to develop;
- anaemia – the oxygen-carrying capacity of the blood is reduced;
- heart failure – inefficient pumping of the blood;
- obesity – fat stored in the abdomen restricts breathing;
- asthma – wheezing with inefficient breathing.

Asthma

Asthma affects the air tubes in the lungs. When a person with asthma comes into contact with something that irritates the air tubes they become narrower because:

- the muscles around the air tubes tighten;
- the lining of the airways becomes inflamed and starts to swell;
- sometimes, sputum (phlegm) builds up.

The result is wheezing, coughing and difficulty in breathing.

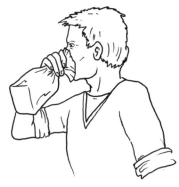

Remedy for hyperventilation
Using a paper bag, breathe slowly in and out 10 times, then breathe without the bag for 15 seconds. Repeat until over-breathing has stopped.

Activity

In your own words, explain how the respiratory and cardiovascular systems work together to supply the cells with oxygen and remove carbon dioxide.

2. **a** Give the difference between inhaling and exhaling.
   b Give examples of various ways of breathing.
   c i What is hyperventilation,
     ii what symptoms can accompany hyperventilation,
     iii what are the symptoms caused by?
   d Give two reasons for temporary breathlessness?
   e What condition can cause chronic breathlessness?
   f i Why does asthma make the air tubes narrower?
     ii Give three symptoms that result.

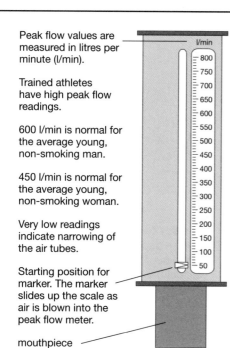

Peak flow values are measured in litres per minute (l/min).

Trained athletes have high peak flow readings.

600 l/min is normal for the average young, non-smoking man.

450 l/min is normal for the average young, non-smoking woman.

Very low readings indicate narrowing of the air tubes.

Starting position for marker. The marker slides up the scale as air is blown into the peak flow meter.

mouthpiece

Peak flow meter

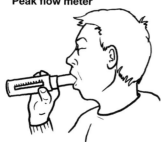

To use a peak flow meter, put the marker at the base of the scale, take a deep breath, place the mouth firmly around the mouthpiece, and make a quick, sharp blow. Do three peak flows and take the highest value. The results can be recorded on a peak flow chart.

Asthma triggers

Asthma triggers are anything that can cause an asthma attack and include:

- **allergens** – substances that irritate the airways, produced for example from house dust mites, animals, pollen and fungal spores;
- **physical and emotional factors** include cold air, chest infections and stress.

Treatment Two types of medicine taken through an inhaler that are often used to control asthma are:

- **preventers** (steroids) prevent asthma developing;
- **relievers** (broncho-dilators) open up the airways and relieve the symptoms of an asthma attack.

Peak flow test

This type of lung function test uses a peak flow meter to measure how quickly air can be blown out of the lungs. It can be used to:

- assess how easily air can be blown out;
- monitor the effectiveness of medical treatment prescribed to relieve the asthma.

Peak flow chart to measure the effect of treatment for asthma

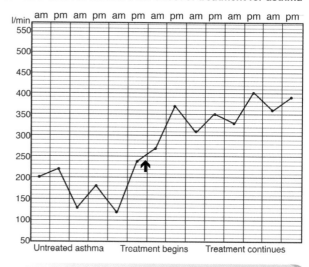

Activities

1. Explain how using a peak flow meter to monitor breathing can indicate the effectiveness of treatment for asthma.
2. Give a talk of at least four minutes on asthma (➲ 'Giving a talk' page 247).
3. Use a questionnaire to find how many people in your class or year group have breathing problems (➲ Questionnaire page 246).

3. a Give examples of asthma triggers.
   b Why may medicines called preventers and relievers be prescribed for asthma?
   c Give two reasons for a peak flow test.
   d i Before using a peak flow meter, where should the marker be,
     ii what makes the marker move up the scale,
     iii what value is recorded on the chart?
   e Are the peak flow values higher in the mornings or evenings?
   f Give the difference between:
     i the first and the last readings on the chart,
     ii the lowest and highest readings on the chart.

Digestive system

The **digestive system** is composed of the **alimentary canal** and various glands attached to it. The **alimentary canal** (the **gut**) is a long tube that extends from mouth to anus. The function of the digestive system is to digest food. As food passes through the alimentary canal it is **digested** (broken down) into very small parts which are absorbed into the blood stream. The waste material from digestion (**faeces, stools**) is eliminated through the anus.

Digestion of food

Salivary glands produce **saliva** – a fluid that keeps the mouth moist, aids the swallowing of food and begins the process of digesting starch.

Liver – the largest gland in the body produces bile that breaks down fat.

Gall bladder – stores bile until it is needed.

Pancreas – a gland that secretes juice which digests carbohydrates, fats and protein.

Intestine wall secretes juice that digests carbohydrates and protein.

Appendix

Rectum – the last part of the large intestine where faeces are stored.

Anus – the hole through which faeces are expelled from the body.

Mouth Teeth chew the food and break it into smaller pieces. It becomes mixed with saliva that begins to break down starch.

Throat (pharynx) pushes food into the gullet.

Gullet (oesophagus) takes food from throat to stomach.

Stomach – a bag in which food is churned up and mixed with gastric juice that continues to break down the food. After a time, the partly digested food gradually passes into the small intestine.

Small intestine – a very long tube where the food mixes with digestive juices from intestine wall, pancreas and liver. These complete the breakdown of food into very small particles which pass through the intestine wall and into the blood stream. The undigested remains pass into the large intestine.

Large intestine (colon) is where excess water from the undigested food is absorbed into the blood stream. The waste matter (**faeces**) passes into the rectum.

Digestive system

1. **a** What is the digestive system composed of?
   b Describe the alimentary canal.
   c Name the six parts of the alimentary canal that food passes through on its way from mouth to anus. Describe what happens to the food in each part.
   d Give a function of:
i saliva,	**ii** liver,
iii gall bladder,	**iv** rectum,
v pancreas,	**vi** intestinal wall.

Activity
a Draw and label a diagram of the digestive system.
b Explain how the structure of the digestive system enables food to be digested.

The mouth

The mouth has several functions. It:

- is the point of entry for food and drink;
- starts the process of digestion by chewing food and mixing it with saliva;
- enables food to be tasted;
- is an air passage to the lungs;
- assists with speech.

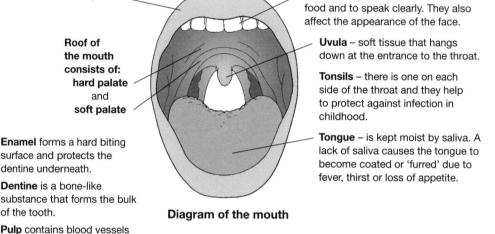

Lips

Teeth are needed to bite and chew food and to speak clearly. They also affect the appearance of the face.

Roof of the mouth consists of:
hard palate
and
soft palate

Uvula – soft tissue that hangs down at the entrance to the throat.

Tonsils – there is one on each side of the throat and they help to protect against infection in childhood.

Tongue – is kept moist by saliva. A lack of saliva causes the tongue to become coated or 'furred' due to fever, thirst or loss of appetite.

Diagram of the mouth

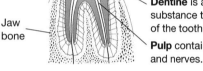

Gum

Jaw bone

Enamel forms a hard biting surface and protects the dentine underneath.

Dentine is a bone-like substance that forms the bulk of the tooth.

Pulp contains blood vessels and nerves.

Section through a molar tooth

Teeth

Teeth are living structures. To build them and keep them healthy, and starting in early childhood, they need:

- enough calcium in the diet;
- fluoride (in drinking water or toothpaste) to strengthen the enamel;
- regular brushing to remove plaque;
- regular dental inspections to identify and treat problems early.

Dental plaque is the soft, sticky layer full of bacteria that continuously forms on the surface of teeth. If plaque is not cleaned off regularly by brushing the teeth, it can absorb calcium from the saliva and form hard **tartar** (**calculus**). Tartar provides shelter for the bacteria in the mouth which produce acids that can damage teeth and gums (➲ next page).

(➲ next page)

Activity

Draw a plan of the teeth of:
i   a young child,
ii an adult.
Colour and label the incisors, canines, premolars and molars to show how the two sets of teeth vary.

---

2. **a** Give five functions of the mouth.
   b Why does the tongue become 'furred'?
   c Why are teeth useful?
   d Describe the three parts of a tooth.
   e **i** Why is fluoride added to drinking water?
      ii Name three other conditions that help to keep teeth healthy.
   f What is dental plaque?
   g **i** What is tartar,
      ii why does it need to be removed?

Care of the teeth

The only structures in the mouth that require care are the teeth:

- Regular and thorough brushing removes plaque and prevents a build-up of calculus;
- Regular inspection and cleaning by a dentist or hygienist will help prevent problems or allow them to be noticed and stopped early.

Gum disease (gingivitis)

Gums infected by bacteria become swollen and sore. Bleeding gums when the teeth are being brushed is usually the first sign of gingivitis. If left untreated, it can develop into **peridontal disease**. This is inflammation of the gum and, if allowed to develop, destroys the tissues (gum and bone) that surround and support the teeth. Gum disease can cause tooth decay.

Tooth decay (caries)

Caries is the decay and crumbling of a tooth and is the most common cause of toothache. Cavities (holes) develop in the teeth and, if the decay reaches the root, it can cause a **root abscess** – a pus-filled swelling in the root of the tooth. **Pus** is a mixture of living and dead bacteria, dead white blood cells and fragments of dead tissue.

Lack of care of the teeth

Teeth that are not cared for can result in:

- toothache;
- losing front teeth – making it difficult to bite food;
- losing back teeth – making it difficult to chew;
- sore gums – gingivitis;
- bad breath (**halitosis**) – unpleasant for other people.

Replacing missing teeth

Missing teeth may be replaced by:

- **dental bridge** – a false tooth that fills the gap caused by a missing tooth. It is permanent and anchored to the teeth on one or both sides.
- **dentures** – artificial teeth that can be removed from the mouth for cleaning. **Denture sore mouth** is inflammation of the gum caused by infection with bacteria when dentures are not regularly cleaned.
- **dental implants** – artificial teeth embedded in the jaw bone are very expensive.

A toothbrush with a large head cleans the surface of the teeth.

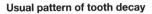

A toothbrush with a small head cleans the sides of the teeth and the edge of the gums.

An interdental toothbrush cleans between the teeth.

Usual pattern of tooth decay

Bacteria in the mouth feed on sugar and produce acids.

The acids dissolve the hard part of the tooth and produce a hole.

This exposes the nerves causing

PAIN

3. **a** What may result from failure to care for the teeth?

   b What is:
   i caries;   ii pus,
   iii a root abscess?

   c How does a root abscess form?

   d Describe the usual pattern of tooth decay.

   e What is;
   i gingivitis,
   ii the first sign of it?

   f i When may peridontal disease develop,
   ii what are the effects?

   g i What are dentures,
   ii what is denture sore mouth?

   h Why use three different types of toothbrush to clean the teeth?

Activity

Give a talk of at least four minutes on 'How to keep teeth healthy'.

Disorders of the digestive system

Cirrhosis
This disease of the liver is usually caused by long-term alcohol abuse. It results in the wasting away of normal liver tissue and its replacement by scar tissue (cirrhosis). If the heavy drinking stops before cirrhosis develops, the liver usually recovers.

Gallstones
These are hard stones that develop in the gall bladder. Usually they are no problem, but may cause indigestion when fat is eaten, or block the bile duct and cause pain and jaundice.

Irritable bowel syndrome (IBS)
The muscles in the wall of the colon tighten up (go into spasm) causing pain with constipation and/or diarrhoea.

Appendicitis is inflammation of the appendix, causing pain.

Crohn's disease causes inflammation in any part of the gut, mostly the small intestine. Typical symptoms include pain and diarrhoea.

Hepatitis
Hepatitis is inflammation of the liver, and is usually due to a virus infection. It causes fever, difficulty in digesting fat, vomiting and **jaundice** (yellowness of the skin and eyes due to increased amounts of bile in the tissues).

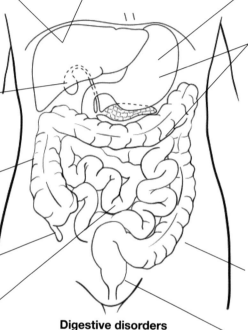

Digestive disorders

Flatulence
Flatulence is due to bubbles of gas in the stomach or intestines. The gas can be air that has been swallowed when gulping food, or it can be produced by bacteria in the large intestine. This results in burping, belching or passing wind (farting).

Heartburn (reflux)
When acid from the stomach flows up into the gullet it causes inflammation and pain. The pain is felt near the heart – hence the name 'heartburn'. Fatty, spicy food can give rise to this condition, especially in people who are overweight.

Gastro-enteritis
This is inflammation of the lining of the stomach (gastritis) and intestines (enteritis), usually due to infection such as food poisoning. The symptoms vary from **nausea** (feeling sick), **vomiting** (being sick) and/or looseness of the bowels (**diarrhoea**) with abdominal pain.

Hernia
A hernia occurs when part of an organ pushes out from where it normally belongs into a neighbouring space. For example, when a part of the intestine pushes through the abdominal wall to lie under the skin in the groin (a **rupture**), or when part of the stomach passes through the diaphragm into the thorax (a **hiatus hernia**).

Piles (haemorrhoids)
These are swollen veins on the inside of the rectum; they are often painful and can bleed.

Activity

a Carry out a media search to find out about a disease of the digestive system.
b Identify the risk factors linked with the disease.
c Describe the care that needs to be given to patients with the disease.
d Explain why this care needs to be given.

4. From the information given above:
   a i Name two disorders that affect the liver and the usual cause of each.
     ii What is jaundice?
   b i Where do gallstones form, ii what may they cause?
   c i Why is 'heartburn' so called, ii when does the pain occur, iii what can give rise to this condition?
   d Describe a hernia.
   e i What is gastro-enteritis?
     ii Give the difference between nausea and vomiting.
   f Name and describe a disorder that affects:
     i the colon, ii appendix, iii rectum.
   g i What causes flatulence, ii where does the gas come from?
   h Describe Crohn's disease.

Diarrhoea

This is the frequent passing of loose, watery faeces. Short-term diarrhoea can be due to food poisoning.

Constipation

Passing hard, dry faeces can be painful, might tear the anus, and can cause bleeding. Constipation can be due to lack of enough fibre from fruit and vegetables in the diet, not drinking enough water, lack of exercise, repeatedly ignoring signals to empty the bowel, repeated use of laxatives or some pain-relievers. Long-term constipation can result in piles.

Laxatives are medicines taken to encourage the bowels to open. A gentle laxative can be taken for a short time, but long-term use can prevent the bowel from functioning normally and can make the person dependent on them (a form of drug dependence).

Indigestion (dyspepsia)

Indigestion is feeling uncomfortable or in pain after eating. There are many causes, but a doctor's advice is needed if indigestion lasts for more than a week, or if it occurs often.

To help prevent indigestion caused by food:

- eat small, regular meals;
- take time to eat slowly and chew food properly;
- avoid very rich (fatty) and spicy foods;
- avoid too much alcohol;
- avoid putting pressure on the stomach by eating hunched forward, or using tight belts or waistbands;
- if indigestion occurs at night, avoid eating or drinking anything for three hours before bedtime.

Indigestion mixtures (antacids) neutralise acid produced by the stomach. Although they give temporary relief from pain caused by acid they:

- do not cure the problem;
- can cause health problems if taken over a long period of time;
- can mask the signs of a serious disorder and therefore should not be taken regularly except on medical advice.

Causes of occasional indigestion
over-eating
eating too quickly
too much rich food
too much alcohol
eating hunched up
eating late at night

Causes of frequent indigestion
heartburn
gallstones
peptic ulcer
hiatus hernia
irritable bowel syndrome

5. a What can short-term diarrhoea be due to?
   b To help prevent constipation, list five actions that a person can take.
   c Why is long-term use of laxatives not recommended?
   d What is indigestion?
   e In two columns, list the causes of occasional indigestion and suggest a way to help prevent each.
   f Name five possible causes of frequent indigestion.
   g i What are antacids?
     ii Give three reasons why long-term use of antacids is not recommended.

Activities

1. Read and summarise information given in two different documents about indigestion.
   • one document explaining the causes of indigestion,
   • the other document advising how to prevent it.
2. In your own words, explain how the digestive and cardio-vascular systems work together to deliver food to the cells.

Urinary system

1. a i What does the urinary tract consist of,
   ii what is its function?
  b Name four parts of the urinary tract.
  c Whereabouts in the body are the kidneys situated?
  d Why can a person manage with one kidney?
  e Give the function of the kidneys, renal arteries, ureters, bladder and urethra.
  f How is urine released from the bladder?
  g Describe incontinence and three of its causes.
  h Calculate how much blood passes through the kidneys in one hour.

Excretion is the removal of waste products from the body:

- The **lungs** excrete carbon dioxide in the air breathed out;
- The **skin** excretes salt and water in sweat;
- The **urinary system** (**renal system**) excretes water, salt, urea, alcohol, drugs, hormones and many other substances in urine.

The **urinary tract** consists of two kidneys, two ureters, a bladder and a urethra.

Kidneys

The kidneys remove waste substances from the body in urine. They do this by filtering the blood as it passes through the kidneys and extracting the waste substances from it together with unwanted water and salt. About 600 ml (1 pint) of blood passes through the kidneys every minute and they are normally so efficient that the body is able to function with only one. This could happen if a kidney is removed because of disease or accident, or is used for transplanting into a close relative.

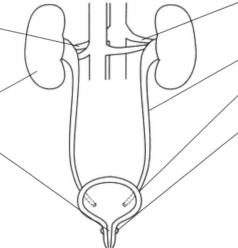

Renal vein removes purified blood from the kidneys.

The two **kidneys** are attached to the back wall of the abdomen above the level of the waist.

Urethra – the tube through which urine leaves the body. In men it is about 20 centimetres long and opens at the end of the penis. In women, it is about 4 cm long and opens into the vulva.

Renal artery carries blood to the kidneys to be purified.

Ureter carries urine to the bladder.

Bladder stores urine.

A **ring of muscle (sphincter)** closes the exit from the bladder. When it relaxes, urine is released and expelled from the body through the urethra. Most people are able to control their bladder and release urine only when they want to.

The urinary system

Incontinence

Incontinence is loss of voluntary control of the bladder and can be due to:

- a leak of urine on coughing or straining (stress incontinence) – this is common in women when the pelvic floor muscles have been weakened by childbirth;
- leakage from a full bladder, common in older men with an enlarged prostate gland;
- dementia (mind loss) when control of the bladder is affected.

Activity

a Draw and label a diagram of the urinary system.
b Explain how the structure of the urinary system enables waste substances to be excreted from the body.

Cystitis

Cystitis is inflammation of the bladder usually caused by an infection. Symptoms are pain in the lower abdomen and the frequent passing of small amounts of urine that stings as it goes through the urethra (urethritis). It is much commoner in women than men.

Kidney stones

These are small stones that form in the kidneys. If they block the flow of urine, or cause infection or severe pain, they can be broken up by shock waves.

Urine

Urine is the watery, yellow fluid produced by the kidneys. The colour can vary. For example, a strong yellow colour implies not drinking enough water and eating beetroot may result in pink urine. Fresh urine usually has little smell unless an infection is present. Stale urine gives off a strong unpleasant smell of ammonia.

Urine tests using a dipstick may be carried out:

- as part of a routine health check;
- to monitor diabetes;
- to screen for infection in the urinary tract;
- to monitor the treatment of a wide range of diseases;
- to check for the illegal use of drugs.

2. a i What is cystitis,
     ii what are the symptoms?
   b i What are kidney stones,
     ii when may they be removed?
   c i Describe urine and its colour.
     ii What makes it smell?
   d Give five reasons for urine tests.
   e Describe a way of testing urine.
   f What substances test positive in urine when a person:
     i is slimming,
     ii has jaundice,
     iii has kidney disease,
     iv may have diabetes,
     v has kidney stones,
     vi may have an infection?

Urine dipstick

	pH	Urine is usually slightly acid
	Glucose	Present in poorly controlled diabetes
	Ketones	Present in slimmers and poorly controlled diabetes
	Protein	Present in urinary tract infection and kidney disease
	Blood	Can indicate kidney stones or urinary tract infection
	Bilirubin	Present in jaundice
	Nitrites	Present in urinary tract infection

Activities

1. Describe a urine test that is carried out as part of a health check.
2. Athletes are banned from taking anabolic steriods. How can they be detected and why are they banned?

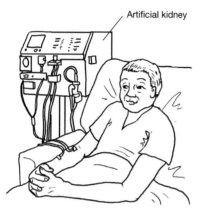

Artificial kidney

Haemodialysis

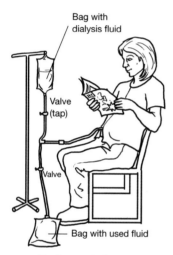

Bag with dialysis fluid

Valve (tap)

Valve

Bag with used fluid

Peritoneal dialysis

Kidney failure

Kidney failure (renal failure) can happen rapidly over days (acute renal failure) or slowly over a period of years (chronic renal failure). Common causes of chronic kidney failure are:

- **Diabetes**. If there is too much glucose in the blood, it can damage the tiny units inside the kidney called nephrons. The nephrons carry out the filtering process, and if they are unable to function, the kidneys will work less well.
- **High blood pressure**. This can put strain on the small blood vessels in the kidneys and damage them.
- **Kidney disease**.

Kidney dialysis

Waste substances need to be removed from the blood because, if they build up, they poison the body. This process is carried out by the kidneys. When the kidneys fail to work properly, the removal of the waste substances can be done by **dialysis**:

- **haemodialysis** uses a machine called an 'artificial kidney' to filter the blood;
- **peritoneal dialysis** uses the lining of the abdomen as a filter.

Haemodialysis

Blood from an artery, usually in the patient's arm, is pumped to the artificial kidney. As the blood passes through the machine, unwanted substances are filtered out. The blood is then returned to a nearby vein. The process can take, for example, four hours three times a week, perhaps in the patient's home if a machine is available for personal use.

Peritoneal dialysis

Fluid flows by gravity from the bag into the patient's abdominal cavity. It is left there for a few hours to give time for waste substances to move from the blood into the fluid. The fluid is then drained off and the process is repeated three or four times a day. The direction in which the fluid flows is controlled by valves.

Activities

1. Find out how kidney dialysis affects patients' lives either by asking a person who is undergoing dialysis or from the media. Write a report of not less than 500 words (➲ Writing a report, page 242; Media search, page 245.)
2. In your own words, explain how the excretory and cardio-vascular systems work together to remove unwanted substances from the body.

3. **a i** Why do waste substances need to be removed from the blood,
    ii what organs in the body carry out this process?
   b What is the difference between acute and chronic kidney failure?
   c Explain why diabetes can cause the kidneys to fail?
   d Why can high blood pressure cause kidney failure?
   e When is dialysis necessary?
   f Name the two types of dialysis.
   g Explain how an artificial kidney works.
   h What happens in peritoneal dialysis?

The nervous system

The nervous system includes the brain, spinal cord and nerves. They form a complicated network of nerve cells (**neurons**) specialised to carry information to and from all parts of the body. The functions of the nervous system include:

- coordination and control of muscle movements;
- receiving information about conditions outside the body from the **sense organs** – eyes, ears, skin, nose and tongue;
- monitoring and controlling conditions inside the body;
- learning from experience and making decisions.

A **trapped nerve in the neck** is due to pressure on a nerve in the neck at the point where it leaves the backbone; it causes pain from the neck down to the wrist.

Lower back pain (lumbago) is mild to severe pain in the lower back which can be acute (short-term) or chronic (long-term).

Sciatica is pain down the leg due to pressure on the **nerves**.

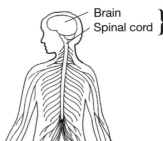

Brain
Spinal cord } **Central nervous system**
If nerve cells in the brain are damaged, as happens with stroke, they cannot be repaired. If the spinal cord is damaged it does not heal.

Nerves carry messages to and from the brain and spinal cord. If a nerve is cut, the ends may grow together, but the nerve fibres may not connect up again in the right way. The part of the body served by the nerve does not then function normally.

Nervous system

Paralysis

Paralysis is loss of muscle power in a part of the body, usually caused by a stroke or injury. **Paraplegia** is paralysis of the lower part of the body due to damage of the spinal cord. The leg muscles cannot function because they are no longer controlled by the brain. There may also be loss of feeling in the legs and disturbed bladder and bowel function. If the spinal cord in the neck is broken the result is **quadriplegia** – paralysis of all four limbs.

Activities

1. Draw and label a diagram of the nervous system.
2. Find out about the effects of paralysis by interviewing, or reading accounts of, people who are paralysed. For example, how the paralysis affects their lifestyle, the equipment they find useful and how much care do they need from the family, carers, the NHS or Social Services. Write a report of your findings and include images. (➲ Writing a report, page 242).

1. a i What does the nervous system consist of,
     ii what are neurons and what do they do?
   b Give four functions of the nervous system.
   c Describe:
     i a trapped nerve in the neck,
     ii lumbago,
     iii sciatica.
   d i What is paralysis,
     ii Why can't a paraplegic walk,
     iii What is quadriplegia?

The brain

The brain is the co-ordinating and decision-making centre of the body. It is composed of millions and millions of nerve cells called neurons (the grey matter of the brain) and nerve fibres (the white matter). The left side of the brain controls the right side of the body, and the right side controls the left side of the body.

Different areas of the brain are responsible for either receiving signals (sensory nerve impulses) from different parts of the body, or sending signals (motor nerve impulses) to the muscles.

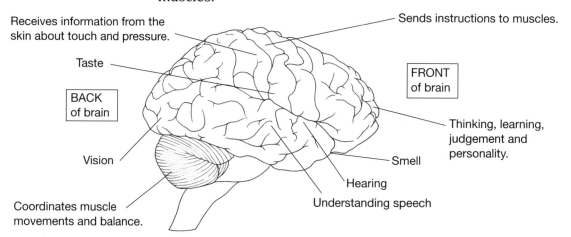

Receives information from the skin about touch and pressure.

Taste

BACK of brain

Vision

Coordinates muscle movements and balance.

Sends instructions to muscles.

FRONT of brain

Thinking, learning, judgement and personality.

Smell

Hearing

Understanding speech

Side view of the brain showing functions of the different areas

| Information from the **sense organs** (eyes, ears, nose, mouth, skin) is sent to the brain. | The brain processes the information and decides how to respond. | Signals are sent to the appropriate muscles to carry out the required actions. |

Decision-making and action in the brain

Headaches

Headaches are very common and have many causes. Most are caused by emotional stress or tiredness and can be relieved by rest and relaxation or a mild pain-reliever (**analgesic**). If a headache lasts for more than a few days, it is advisable to see a doctor. A **migraine** is a headache, often on only one side, that lasts from a few hours to a day or longer. It may begin with an 'aura' (flashing lights, etc.) and is often accompanied by nausea, vomiting and the dislike of bright light.

Activity

Explain how the structure of the nervous system enables it to carry out its functions.

2. **a** What does the brain do and what is it composed of?
   b Draw a simple diagram of the brain and label the functions of the different parts.
   c Describe the actions that take place in the brain when a car driver sees and avoids a pedestrian.
   d i What are two common causes of a headache,
      ii what can help to relieve a headache,
      iii When should a doctor be consulted?
   e Give some symptoms of migraine.

Learning disabilities

A **learning disability** (**learning difficulty**) is a limited ability to learn and communicate. The disability may be mild, moderate or severe and can be caused by:

- **incomplete development of the brain** (developmental disability) due to:
  - a genetic disorder, for example Down's syndrome,
  - infection in the womb, for example by rubella,
  - birth injuries, for example cerebral palsy,
- **infection that affects the brain**, for example a complication of meningitis;
- **brain damage**, for example by a road traffic accident.

Autism

Autism is a disorder that develops in early childhood. People with autism:

- **find it difficult to communicate with others** – they do not understand other people's facial expressions, tone of voice or gestures;
- **do not show emotions** such as love and affection – sometimes the only emotion is occasional outbursts of rage;
- **do not understand other people's feelings**, so find it difficult to make friends;
- **find it difficult to use imagination** – they have a limited range of activities that are carried out rigidly, and there is resistance to any changes in daily routine and familiar surroundings.

These difficulties may make autistic children slow learners and about 50 per cent have learning disabilities. But some are very intelligent and may be gifted in certain areas, for example in music, art or arithmetic.

Asperger's syndrome This is a less severe form of autism. There may be a limited ability to communicate orally, a lack of common sense and persistence in following particular routines (obsessive behaviour). Although people with this condition are aware of their disability, they often find it very difficult to make friends.

3. **a** What is a learning disability?
   b i What is a developmental disability?
   ii Give three possible causes for this condition.
   iii Give two other causes for a learning disability.
   c When does autism develop?
   d Describe four characteristics of autism.
   e Are all people with autism slow learners? Explain.
   f Describe Asperger's syndrome.

Activities

1. **a** Research the facilities available for education and training in your area for children and adults with learning disabilities or autism. Add them to the map of your area recommended on page 4.
   b Give a talk of at least four minutes on your research.
2. Revise the rights of people with disabilities (➲ page 85).

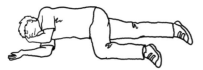

Recovery position
This is the recommended position for all unconscious people, for example following an epileptic fit.

4. a i What is meningitis,
  ii what causes the disease,
  iii what are the symptoms?
  b i What are the signs of epilepsy?
  ii Describe a major epileptic fit.
  iii Describe the recovery position.
  c Name three progressive disorders of the nervous system.
  d In which of the disorders named in **c**:
  i do the muscles lose strength,
  ii are movements uncoordinated,
  iii do the muscles become stiff,
  iv may the eyes be affected,
  v may start at an early age,
  vi is the speech affected, not the mind?
  e What is encephalitis?

Disorders of the nervous system

Meningitis

Meningitis is inflammation of the membranes covering the brain and spinal cord. It is caused by infection with viruses or, less often but more seriously, bacteria. Unless quickly diagnosed and treated, death can occur rapidly, particularly in children.

Encephalitis

Encephalitis is inflammation of brain tissue caused, for example, by infection with bacteria or viruses.

Multiple sclerosis (MS)

This is a progressive disease of the central nervous system caused when small scattered patches of nerve cells fail to work. The disease comes and goes and the symptoms depend on which parts of the brain and spinal cord are affected: perhaps blurred vision, uncoordinated movements, unsteady walking and slurred speech. MS usually starts between the ages of 20 and 50.

Epilepsy

Signs of epilepsy are fits (**seizures**) and the temporary loss of consciousness. In a major epileptic fit, the person loses consciousness, falls to the ground, makes jerking movements which gradually ease, then goes into a deep sleep.

Motor neurone disease (MND)

This disorder causes progressive weakness of the muscles and they eventually stop working. It does not affect the mind or other body systems, and occurs most commonly after the age of 50.

Parkinson's disease

This is a progressive condition of the part of the brain that controls the muscles. Stiffness and **tremor** (shaking) of the muscles makes movements slow and clumsy, these symptoms usually appearing after the age of 50. Muscles used for speaking are also affected, making speech slow and delivered in a dull monotone.

Activity

Find out more about meningitis and septicaemia from, for example, the Meningitis Trust. Write a leaflet for carers describing the signs and symptoms, the Glass Test and what to do in a medical emergency.

Mental illness

Mental illness is being unable to cope with every-day life for weeks, months or years at a time. It affects all aspects of life – sleep, work and relationships. Sadness, anxiety and fear are a part of life's experiences for everyone but they only become a mental illness when they are severe, long-term and affect the person's social life.

Most mental illness can be treated or controlled either by counselling or by medication. When a short stay in psychiatric hospital is necessary, it may be followed by visits from the community psychiatric nurse or social worker.

Mental disorders

It is estimated that about one in four people are mentally ill at some point in their lives, mainly with one of the following conditions.

Depression Extreme sadness and feelings of being hopeless, helpless and unable to cope are symptoms of depression. It has been described as like falling into a big black hole with no way out. There is no interest in other people or their activities. Often the patient feels very tired and suffers from **insomnia** (inability to sleep). Sufferers are aware of their abnormal behaviour but are unable to control it. **Post-natal depression** is a severe form of depression that follows childbirth. It is far more serious and long-term than the 'baby blues' (mild depression) that can occur as the mother's hormones settle down.

Bipolar disorder (previously known as manic depression) is a disorder in which behaviour swings between extreme depression and extreme over-activity (mania).

Anxiety A person with this condition becomes so anxious about trivial things that their normal life is seriously affected. It can cause fainting, dizziness, breathlessness and poor concentration.

Obsessive-compulsive disorder (OCD) This is marked by repeatedly performing actions (compulsions), for example hand-washing, to relieve the anxiety caused by recurring thoughts (obsessions), for example the fear of germs.

5. **a i** What is mental illness,
   ii how can it effect a person's life,
   iii how is most mental illness treated?
   b What is bipolar disorder and what was it formerly called?
   c i Give some symptoms of depression,
   ii are the sufferers aware of their behaviour?
   d Compare postnatal depression with the 'baby blues'.
   e When does anxiety become a mental illness?
   f i What does OCD stand for?
   ii Explain the difference between an obsession and a compulsion.

Activity

Find statistics from the internet that agree or disagree with the statement 'About one in four people are mentally ill at some point in their lives'. (➲ Media search page 245.)

Phobia A phobia is an extreme fear of a particular thing or event that is so strong it restricts the person's life. Examples are **agoraphobia** (fear of open spaces), **claustrophobia** (fear of enclosed spaces) or **arachnophobia** (fear of spiders).

Addiction

An addiction is a habit that has become impossible to break. Common addictions are to alcohol and some drugs. The usual treatment aims at the gradual withdrawal of the cause of the addiction and eventually total abstinence.

Schizophrenia

People with this condition lose contact with reality. They withdraw into a private, unreal world with **delusions** (mistaken beliefs) and **hallucinations** (seeing and hearing things that are not there). The illness usually starts in young adults and the right treatment can result in long periods of normal behaviour.

Dementia (mind loss)

Dementia is loss of normal mental ability. It usually occurs gradually with symptoms that include loss of memory, confusion, and changes in personality and behaviour. The most common form is **Alzheimer's disease** – a progressive disease of the brain. Although most people who develop dementia are over the age of 60, it is not a normal part of growing old, and most older people never develop dementia.

Coping with dementia is distressing for both the patient and the family carers. The patient tends to behave in ways that other people find more and more irritating or upsetting; the patient does not understand why. When family members struggle to cope with the continuous and demanding job of caring, they may become physically and emotionally worn out. It is important that their own health is safe-guarded so that they can continue to care. The solution may be day care or respite care for the patient to give the family a break.

Activity

From the website of the Alzheimer's Society, in the section 'Caring for someone with dementia', select 10 points that you consider important for a carer to know.

6. **a i** What is a phobia?
   ii Explain the difference between agoraphobia and claustrophobia.
   b What is an addiction and what is the usual treatment?
   c Describe schizophrenia.
   d i What is dementia,
   ii what are its effects,
   iii what is the most common form,
   iv is dementia a normal part of growing old? Explain.
   e Explain why dementia is distressing for family carers.
   f Why is day care or respite care for people with dementia very important for their family carers?

Treating mental illness

GPs treat milder forms of depression and anxiety by talking with the patients, and sometimes prescribing medicines such as anti-depressants. Those with severe mental illness are referred to a psychiatrist, a psychologist or trained counsellors.

Psychiatrists are doctors who specialise in the study and treatment of mental disorders. Being medically trained, they are able to prescribe medicines as part of the treatment.

Psychologists study normal and abnormal behaviour and are trained to assess and treat the mentally ill. **Educational psychologists** advise on the management of children.

Psychotherapists help people to understand their difficulties, weaknesses and anxieties in order to manage them. They generally treat the more complex problems that have built up over many years. **Psychiatric hospitals** have clinics and beds for in-patients who will be cared for by psychiatric nurses. When discharged, patients may receive care from a community psychiatric nurse.

Cognitive behavioural therapy (CBT) helps patients to change how they think ('cognition') and what they do ('behaviour'). Therapists work with patients suffering from sleeping difficulties, relationship problems, drug and alcohol abuse, depression, anxiety and phobias.

Working with a therapist, the patient looks for explanations for the distressing events in their life. To help this process, the patient may be asked to keep a diary. The diary is then used to identify the pattern of thoughts, emotions, bodily feelings and actions. This makes it easier to see how they are connected, and how the patient can best deal with them. After a course of therapy, the patient should have developed the skills to cope on their own with any negative events that occur in the future.

Activity

Research the facilities available in your own area for people with, or recovering from, mental disorders or mental illness.

---

7. **a** When a GP diagnoses mental illness, what treatment might the patient receive?
   b What is the difference between a psychiatrist, a psychologist, and an educational psychologist?
   c **i** What is psychotherapy?
      ii Describe a psychiatric hospital.
   d **i** What is CBT,
      ii why is CBT used,
      iii which patients might be offered CBT?
   e Why may patients undergoing CBT be asked to keep a diary?

The eyes

The **eyes** are the organs of sight. Their function is to receive light rays and send the information to the brain. Each eye consists of a three-layered eyeball filled with clear jelly and, in the front part, watery fluid and other structures. The eyes are set in sockets in the skull and protected by eyebrows, eyelids and eyelashes. Muscles attached to the eyeball move it to look in different directions.

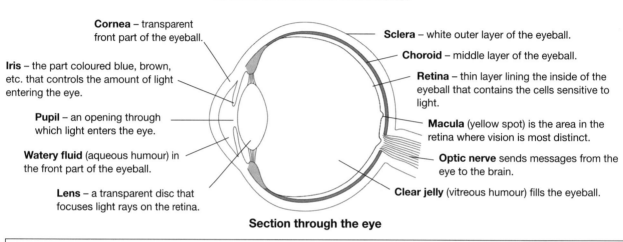

Cornea – transparent front part of the eyeball.

Iris – the part coloured blue, brown, etc. that controls the amount of light entering the eye.

Pupil – an opening through which light enters the eye.

Watery fluid (aqueous humour) in the front part of the eyeball.

Lens – a transparent disc that focuses light rays on the retina.

Sclera – white outer layer of the eyeball.

Choroid – middle layer of the eyeball.

Retina – thin layer lining the inside of the eyeball that contains the cells sensitive to light.

Macula (yellow spot) is the area in the retina where vision is most distinct.

Optic nerve sends messages from the eye to the brain.

Clear jelly (vitreous humour) fills the eyeball.

Section through the eye

Causes of blindness

Cataract – the lens becomes cloudy, making it difficult to see. Sight can be restored by removing the lens and replacing it with a plastic lens.

Diabetes can damage the retina.

Detached retina – the retina becomes loose and vision is lost from the affected area.

Macular degeneration – loss of function of the central part of the retina, and the most common cause of blindness in the elderly.

Glaucoma occurs when too much pressure builds up in the eyeball, causing pain, blurred vision and, if not treated, blindness. Treatment to reduce the fluid is by eye drops, tablets or surgery.

1. a i Describe the position of the eyes in the skull,
   ii How does an eyeball move?
   b Describe the:
   i cornea,   ii pupil,
   iii iris,   iv lens,
   v retina,   vi optic nerve.
   c i What is the eyeball filled with?
   ii What causes glaucoma,
   iii how is it treated?
   d i What causes a cataract,
   ii how is it treated?
   e Name three causes of blindness associated with the retina.
   f Why do children need to have their eyes tested?
   g Why are eye tests recommended for adults

Care of the eyes

Eye-strain Working in a poor light or not wearing glasses when they are needed results in tired eyes and headaches. Permanent damage to eyesight is unlikely.

Eye checks are advised for:

- **children** because short sight or long sight can develop if the eyes grow out of shape. Poor vision affects school work, behaviour and physical activities.
- **adults**, especially when there is a family history of eye disorders. Disorders can be discovered by looking inside the eyes before any symptoms have appeared.
- **diabetics**, diabetes can affect the eyes and be the cause of blindness if not treated early.

Activities

1. Draw a simple diagram of a section through the eye. Describe its function and each part.
2. Trachoma is the commonest cause of blindness world wide. What causes it, how is it treated and how can it be prevented?

Vision

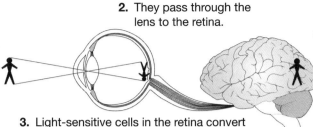

1. Light rays enter the eye.

2. They pass through the lens to the retina.

3. Light-sensitive cells in the retina convert them into messages that are sent along the optic nerve to the brain.

4. When the messages reach the part of the brain concerned with vision, they are converted into images (pictures).

Vision (eyesight, sight) is the ability to see

Visual impairment

Visual impairment is the reduction of the ability to see and includes short-sightedness, long-sightedness, astigmatism and blindness. Most people with a visual impairment need to wear glasses or contact lenses.

Causes of visual impairment include:

- a birth defect, for example rubella damage in the womb;
- eye injury, for example accidents or sun damage during an eclipse;
- a disorder that develops, for example, cataract or glaucoma;
- diseases such as diabetes and trachoma;
- damage to the part of the brain concerned with vision by, for example, a stroke.

Blindness

This is the absence of useful sight. Most blind people have some awareness of light, but their sight is very poor. People with very poor sight are registered with Social Services as either:

- **blind** – they are unable to perform any actions for which eyesight is essential.
- **partially sighted** – this means that the person's eyesight is so poor that it is a handicap to daily life.

Colour 'blindness'

Colour blindness is the inability to distinguish certain colours. It is an inherited condition. The most common form affects males who are unable to distinguish red from green.

2. a Explain the difference between vision and visual impairment.

b Use the diagram above to explain how we are able to see.

c i What is blindness,
ii who registers blind people,
iii is it usual for a blind person to be totally blind,
iv what are the two categories of blindness?

d Describe five causes of blindness.

e i What is colour blindness,
ii what is the most common form?

Activities

1. The RNIB supports blind and partially sighted people. Find out from their website what training, services and support they offer. Summarise the information in at least 500 words.
2. Interview a person who is blind. Find out how their daily life is affected and how difficulties are overcome.
3. What are the differences between an optician, an optometrist and an ophthalmologist? What training is required for each of these careers?

The Ears

The ears have two functions: hearing and balance. Each ear has three parts. The **outer ear** contains the visible part (pinna) and the ear canal. The ear drum separates the outer ear from the middle ear. The delicate parts – middle and inner ear – are well protected inside the bone of the skull. The **middle ear** is a cavity containing three small bones (**ossicles**). The **inner ear** consists of the **cochlea**, which contains the sensory cells for hearing, and the **semicircular canals** which contain those for balance.

How we hear

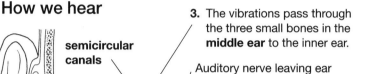

1. The **ear lobe (pinna)** directs sound waves into the ear canal.

2. The sound waves strike the **ear drum** and make it vibrate.

3. The vibrations pass through the three small bones in the **middle ear** to the inner ear.

4. Vibrations cause the **sensory cells** in the **cochlea** in the inner ear to send impulses (messages) along the **auditory nerve** to the brain.

5. When the impulses reach the area of the **brain** concerned with hearing they are interpreted as sounds.

Labels on diagram: semicircular canals; Auditory nerve leaving ear; Eustachian tube

1. a Name the two functions of the ear.
   b Which part of the ear is concerned with balance?
   c Describe the outer, middle and inner parts of the ear.
   d How are the delicate parts of the ear protected?
   e Describe the chain of events (1–5) that enables us to hear.
   f What is the function of the Eustachian tube?
   g Complete the chart on the causes of deafness.

Part	Cause of deafness
Ear canal	

Activity

Draw a diagram of a section through the ear. Label and describe the function of each part.

Causes of deafness

Hearing depends on the chain of events 1-5 described above and damage or disorder to any part in the chain results in deafness. For example:

- a build-up of **wax** in the ear canal forms a barrier to the entry of sound waves;
- a **perforated ear drum** (with a hole in it) stops it vibrating properly;
- **glue ear** – sticky fluid in the middle ear following infection stops the ossicles from vibrating properly;
- **damage to the sensory cells** in the cochlea reduces messages to the brain. Damage is caused by very loud noise. These cells also decay as part of the natural process of ageing;
- **damage to the auditory nerve** stops messages from the ear reaching the brain;
- **damage to the part of the brain concerned with hearing** stops messages from the ear being heard;
- **blocked Eustachian tubes** can be caused by a build up of mucus, as happens with a cold. The Eustachian tubes connect the middle ear with the throat and allow air pressure on both sides of the eardrum to equalise.

Types of deafness

Deafness, 'hearing impairment' or 'hearing loss' means that there is a problem with one or both ears that affects hearing. The deafness can be total, partial, temporary, permanent or gradual.

- **Total deafness** means no sounds can be heard in that ear; it is rare for a person to be totally deaf in both ears.
- **Partial deafness** is much more common. Some sounds are heard but not others; this makes it difficult for a deaf person to understand what other people are saying.
- **Temporary deafness** can be due to:
- a build-up of wax in the outer ear;
- a middle ear infection;
- a blocked Eustachian tube which doesn't allow the pressures to equalise on both sides of the ear drum – this can occur when going quickly down a steep hill in a car or taking off in an aeroplane.
  Note: Normal hearing returns when the wax is removed, the infection cured, or when pressure across the ear drum is equalised.
- **Permanent deafness** results from damage to parts of the ear, the auditory nerve, or the part of the brain responsible for hearing.
- **Gradual loss of hearing** occurs from adolescence onwards. Most older people are unable to hear as well as they used to, especially high-pitched sounds. Hearing loss is increased by noise such as loud music or machinery.

Tinnitus

Tinnitus is ringing, buzzing or whistling sounds in the ear. It may be caused by continuous exposure to loud noise or by infection. It can occur naturally with increasing age.

Balance

The body remains in a balanced position due to the three fluid-filled semicircular canals. Whenever the head moves, the sensory cells in the canals detect movement in the fluid they are bathed in. This information is sent along the auditory nerve to the brain, and the brain responds by sending messages to the appropriate muscles to keep the body balanced. **Dizziness** can be due to spinning the body, turning the head quickly or by inflammation of the inner ear.

2. **a** What is a hearing impairment?
   b Explain the difference between total and partial deafness.
   c Which type of deafness:
   i happens as people get older,
   ii can be due to brain damage,
   iii is rare in both ears,
   iv can disappear?
   d Give three causes of temporary deafness.
   e Describe tinnitus and its causes.
   f How does the body keep itself in an upright position?
   g Give three causes of dizziness.

Activity

The RNID is an organisation for people who are deaf or hard of hearing. Find out from their website what training, services and support they offer. Summarise the information in at least 500 words.

Reproductive systems

Male reproductive system

The male reproductive system is situated in the lower part of the abdomen. It has three functions:

- makes the male hormone testosterone;
- makes sperm;
- ejects semen into the vagina of the female, essential to produce new individuals and the survival of the human race.

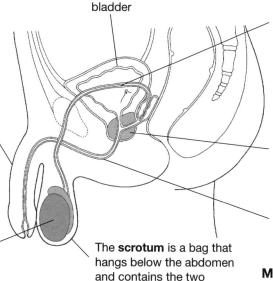

bladder

The **penis** is used for both urination and reproduction. The **foreskin** covers and protects the tip of the penis. **Circumcision** is the removal of the foreskin by surgery, and is carried out by some religious groups. Its removal can reduce the spread of HIV (the cause of AIDS).

The two **testes** (each is a **testis**) begin to produce sperm during puberty and continue to do so throughout life, although the quantity becomes less in older men.

Vas deferens (sperm tube) carries sperm away from the testis to the urethra. **Vasectomy** is an operation in which the sperm tubes are cut and the ends sealed. It causes sterility and is a method of contraception.

Prostate gland secretes fluid that is mixed with sperm to form semen – a thick, milky-white fluid.

Urethra carries both semen and urine to outside the body.

The **scrotum** is a bag that hangs below the abdomen and contains the two testes (**testicles**).

Male reproductive system (side view)

Disorders

The **prostate gland** surrounds the outlet from the bladder. From middle age onwards, it enlarges. This may cause a frequent desire to urinate, difficulty in doing so and a poor stream of urine. Treatment is by surgery to remove the gland or by medicines that shrink it.

Sterility (infertility) means unable to have children.

Impotence is the inability to maintain an erection sufficient to have sexual intercourse.

1. **a** Name the three functions of the male reproductive system.
   b Which of the parts:
   i make sperm,
   ii transport sperm to the penis,
   iii contains the testes,
   iv protects the tip of the penis and what name is given to its removal?
   c Name the two functions of the penis.
   d Explain why the prostate gland may need treatment?
   e Give the difference between sterility and impotence.
   f i What is vasectomy,
   ii Why is it carried out?

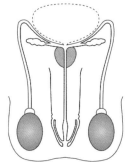

Male reproductive system (front view)

Activity

a Copy the diagram on the left. Then, using the diagram above as a guide, label:
penis   prostate gland   scrotum
vas deferens   testis
urethra   foreskin   bladder
b Explain how the structure of the male reproductive system enables it to carry out its functions.

Female reproductive system

The female reproductive system is situated in the lower part of the abdominal cavity. Its functions are to:

- make the female hormones that control the development and functioning of the female organs, breasts, periods and pubic hair;
- make eggs;
- receive sperm;
- protect and feed an unborn child;
- give birth.

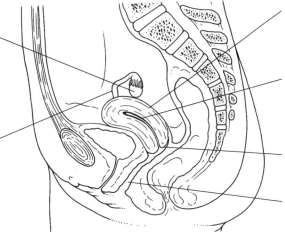

The **ovaries** produce hormones and eggs. One egg (sometimes more) is released each month from one of the ovaries.

The **Fallopian tube** (oviduct; egg tube) takes eggs from the ovary to the uterus; fertilisation takes place in the Fallopian tube.

The **uterus** (womb) is made of muscle and enlarges as the baby develops during pregnancy.

The **uterus lining** (endometrium) is shed every month during a period if an egg is not fertilised.

The **cervix** (neck of the uterus).

The **vagina** is a muscular tube and the place where sperm are deposited during intercourse.

Female reproductive system (side view)

Disorders

Fibroids are lumps that develop in the wall of the uterus. They often cause pain and excessive menstrual bleeding. They may become very large and, although not cancerous, may need to be removed.

Hysterectomy is an operation to remove the womb. There are a number of medical reasons for its removal.

Cervical cancer is cancer of the cervix, a common type of cancer in women. It can be detected before it develops by regular cervical smear tests.

> ## Activity
>
> **a** Copy the diagram on the right. Then, using the diagram above as a guide, label:
> ovaries   Fallopian tubes   uterus
> uterus lining   cervix   vagina.
> **b** Explain how the structure of the female reproductive system enables it to carry out its functions.

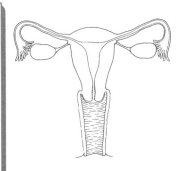

Female reproductive system (front view)

2. **a** **i** Where are the female organs situated?
   ii Name five functions.
   b Which part of the female reproductive system:
   i produces eggs,
   ii produces hormones,
   iii receives sperm,
   iv is where fertilisation takes place,
   v is where a baby develops,
   vi is shed during a period.
   c **i** What are fibroids,
   ii why may they be removed?
   d What is a hysterectomy?
   e What is the purpose of cervical smear tests?

Endocrine system

The **endocrine system** consists of endocrine glands that produce hormones. A **hormone** is a substance produced in one part of the body and carried in the blood stream to affect another part of the body. Although hormones travel to all parts of the body, each only affects certain tissues or organs called **target organs**.

When endocrine glands become over-active or under-active, health problems occur. An example is the thyroid gland:

- an **over-active thyroid** produces too much hormone, causing excessive effects on the body;
- an **under-active thyroid** does not produce enough hormone to keep the body functioning properly.

The **thyroid gland** in the front of the neck. It produces:
- **thyroid hormone** – controls the rate at which the chemical activities occur inside the cells (the metabolic rate).

The **adrenal glands** are situated one above each kidney. They produce:
- **adrenaline** – prepares the body for action (fight or flight);
- **corticosteroids** (commonly called 'steroids') are essential for many processes.

The **ovaries** are in the lower abdomen of females. They produce:
- **oestrogen** – controls the development and functioning of the female sex organs;
- **progesterone** – the pregnancy hormone.

The **pituitary gland** is attached to the underside of the brain. It produces hormones that control other endocrine glands. It also produces:
- **growth hormone** that stimulates the growth of bones and muscles;
- **prolactin** that stimulates the breasts to produce milk;
- **oxytocin** that stimulates the uterus to contract at the end of pregnancy.

The **pancreas** is in the abdomen behind the stomach. It produces:
- **insulin** – reduces the level of sugar (glucose) in the blood;
- **glucagon** – raises the level of sugar (glucose) in the blood.

The two **testes** in males (each is a testis) are situated below the abdomen. They produce:
- **testosterone** – controls the development and functioning of the male sex organs.

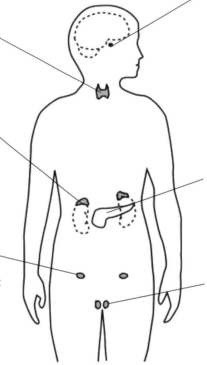

Endocrine glands and hormones

Activity

Find out: **i** why all babies are given a thyroid function test, **ii** the effects in an adult of an overactive thyroid, an underactive thyroid, and the treatments that may be given. Write up your findings in two different documents, one document being at least 500 words long.

1. **a** What is the endocrine system?
   b What is a hormone?
   c What are 'target organs'?
   d What happens when endocrine glands malfunction? Give an example.
   e Copy and complete the table below.

Gland	Position in body	Hormone(s)	Function of hormone

Homeostasis

Homeostasis means maintaining a steady state. Although the conditions outside the body are constantly changing, it is essential for conditions inside the body to remain steady. The millions of cells in the body can only function well and stay healthy when the conditions are kept within narrow limits. Too great a change in any one of them leads to ill-health. Conditions that need to be kept within limits include body temperature, blood glucose levels, hormone levels and levels of oxygen and carbon dioxide.

Regulation of body temperature

The temperature inside the body is maintained at about 37°C as the amount of heat produced in the body is continually balanced by the amount of heat being lost.

When the body is too hot:

- **heat is lost as:**
  – **blood vessels in the skin dilate** (enlarge). This allows more blood to flow into the skin. Heat from the blood is then radiated away into the air (if air temperature is below 37°C).
  – **sweat glands make more sweat**. This flows out onto the skin, and heat is lost from the body as the sweat evaporates.
  – **air movement is increased**, for example by fanning yourself.
- **less heat is produced** as movements become slower or stop.

When the body is too cold:

- **heat loss from the body is reduced** as
  – blood vessels in the skin shut down,
  – sweat glands become inactive,
- **more heat is produced** by movements such as shivering, swinging the arms and stamping the feet.

Maintaining a constant body temperature

When the body is too hot...

sweat　　　heat

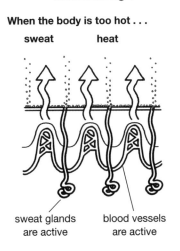

sweat glands　　blood vessels
are active　　　are active

As body temperature falls...

heat

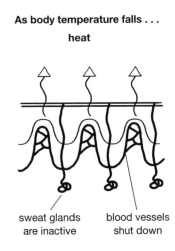

sweat glands　　blood vessels
are inactive　　shut down

1. **a i** Explain the meaning of homeostasis,
   ii Why do conditions inside the body need to remain steady?
   iii Name four conditions.
   b When the body is too hot, what happens to the:
   i blood vessels in the skin,
   ii sweat glands?
   c When the body is too cold, what happens to the:
   i blood vessels in the skin,
   ii sweat glands?

135

Maintaining blood glucose (sugar) levels

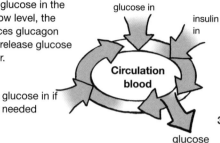

1. Glucose from food in the gut enters the blood stream.

glucose in

insulin in

2. A high glucose level stimulates the pancreas to produce insulin into the blood stream.

4. If the amount of glucose in the blood falls to a low level, the pancreas produces glucagon (➲ page 134) to release glucose stored in the liver.

Circulation blood

glucose in if needed

glucose out

3. The insulin causes the cells in liver to take up excess glucose from the blood for storage.

Diabetes is caused by a shortage of insulin in the blood.

A shortage of insulin means that cells cannot absorb sugar out of the blood.

This results in a high level of glucose remaining in the blood.

Some of the glucose is excreted in the urine, taking water with it.

The individual is then very thirsty and drinks much more water than usual.

Diabetes

Diabetes is a common condition where the level of glucose (sugar) in the blood is too high. There are two types, 1 and 2. **Type 1 diabetes** occurs mainly in young people and develops rapidly. Insulin production stops almost completely causing weight loss, tiredness and thirst.

Type 2 diabetes develops more slowly when the body becomes resistant to the insulin it produces. The symptoms are similar to those of Type 1 diabetes. Type 2 diabetes is common mainly in middle or old age; also in people who are overweight with a large waist measurement and who have a family history of diabetes. It is becoming more common in younger people because of increasing obesity.

People with uncontrolled diabetes are at risk from damage to their heart, circulation, eyesight, kidney failure, heart attacks, stroke, and gangrene in their feet that can result in amputation. It is therefore important to keep blood glucose levels as normal as possible.

Treatment for diabetes

- **Diet** People with diabetes should (like everyone else) aim to eat a balanced diet that is low in fat (especially saturated fat), salt and sugar, and high in fibre (fruit, vegetables, pulses). Special diabetic foods are not needed. (➲ page 233 Diet.)
- **Physical activity** – any type of moderate exercise that is regular and enough to give slight shortness of breath.
- **Tablets** to lower blood glucose levels when the condition cannot be controlled by diet alone.
- **Insulin** by injection to lower blood glucose levels for Type 1 and some Type 2.

2. a Draw a diagram to show how the blood sugar is controlled.
   b What is diabetes?
   c Explain why thirst is usually a symptom of diabetes.
   d Name the two types of diabetes.
   e Which type of diabetes:
     i occurs mainly in older people,
     ii why is it becoming more common in younger people?
   f What can uncontrolled diabetes result in?
   g Describe the types of treatment available for diabetes.

Activities

1. Suggest at least 10 foods suitable for diabetics and 10 unsuitable foods.
2. Is the incidence of diabetes increasing or decreasing? Explain how you reached your conclusion. (➲ Media search page 245.)

Blood pressure (see also page 107)

The function of blood pressure is to move blood around the body from arteries to capillaries to veins so that the circulation can distribute substances such as oxygen, food and hormones to the tissues. Blood pressure varies constantly during the day, rising when the body is active or anxious, and falling back to a lower level when the body is at rest.

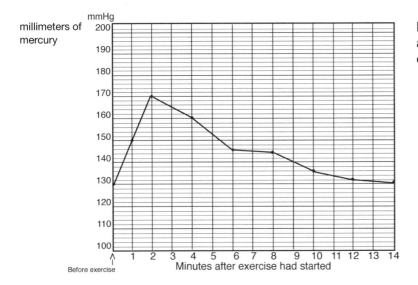

Blood pressure (systolic) of a man who has run up and down 3 flights of stairs

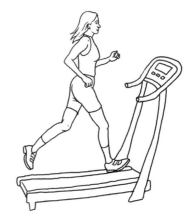

Maintaining oxygen levels

The body needs a constant supply of oxygen to release energy in the cells (from glucose). Energy is required for the chemical processes that keep the cells alive, including those needed to keep the body warm and moving. The amount of oxygen needed at any particular time depends on the amount of activity taking place. The oxygen supply is maintained by the rate and depth of breathing:

- the **rate of breathing** is the number of breaths per minute;
- the **depth of breathing** is the amount of air inhaled per breath. The rate and depth of breathing depend on age, the level of fitness, and whether the person is resting or active.

3. **a** Describe the function of blood pressure.
   b Why does blood pressure vary?
   c **i** How long does it take for the BP to return to the resting level,
   ii how long does it take for the BP to return half way back to resting level?
   d **i** Why does the body need energy,
   ii what is the energy used for,
   iii how much oxygen is required,
   iv how is the oxygen supply adjusted?
   e What does the rate and depth of breathing depend on?

Activity

At rest, a fit young woman took about 16 breaths a minute and inhaled about half a litre (0.5 of a litre) of air with each breath. With hard exercise, she increased the amount of air she breathed each minute to 80 litres. Using this information, calculate:

i how much air she breathed per minute at rest;
ii how much more air per minute she breathed when exercising hard than when she was at rest.

Disease

1. a i What are pathogens,
   ii where are they
       found?
   b How does the body help
       prevent infectious
       disease:
       i on the skin (two
           ways),
       ii on the eyes,
       iii in the airways,
       iv in the blood stream,
       v in food and drink?
   c i Why do infectious
           diseases occur,
       ii Which three groups
           have less resistance
           to disease?
   d Copy and complete the
       chart.

Type of disease	Cause	Examples
Infection		

A **disease** is an illness or disorder of the body. It may be:

- **infection** due to germs, mainly bacteria and viruses, for example salmonella and influenza;
- **cancer** due to uncontrolled cell growth, for example lung cancer and leukaemia;
- **failure of a body part** due to malfunction, for example heart attack and dementia;
- **auto-immune** disorders which occur when the body attacks its own tissues, such as asthma and rheumatoid arthritis;
- **inherited** when an abnormal gene is passed on from parent to child, for example, cystic fibrosis and haemophilia;
- **congenital** when it is present at birth, for example cerebral palsy and congenital dislocation of the hip;
- **mental disorder** when the emotions and behaviour are affected, for example depression and schizophrenia.

Infectious disease

Bacteria and other microbes are too small to be seen with the naked eye but they are everywhere – air, water, soil, food. Some are beneficial, most are harmless and a few, called **germs** (pathogens), can cause disease. Fortunately the body has defences against them known as 'barriers to infection'.

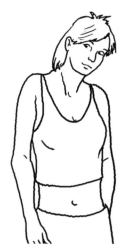

The **skin** is a protective covering to the body and protects against entry of germs.

Acid in the stomach destroys germs that enter the body in food and drink.

Blood clots and scabs over cuts and wounds prevent the entry of germs into the skin.

Tears keep the eyeball moist and contain a substance that destroys germs.

Mucous membrane lining the mouth and airways produces mucus that traps germs and dust in air that is inhaled.

White blood cells and antibodies circulate around the body in the blood stream, and attack any germs that they come across.

Barriers to infection

Activity

Write two documents, one of which should be more than 500 words long, on 'The body's barriers to infection' and 'Preventing infection'. (➲ page 242.)

Infectious diseases occur when the body's defences are unable to prevent the entry of germs or to destroy them. Healthy young adults have more resistance to disease than:

- those in poor health;
- young children who have not had time to build up enough immunity after breast-feeding has ceased;
- elderly people whose 'barriers to infection' have become less efficient.

Cancer

Cancer is a disorder of cell growth. Most cells in the body are capable of growing and dividing into two to produce new cells, either to increase the size of the body or to replace old worn-out cells. Normal cells know when to stop dividing, but when cells multiply in an uncontrolled way they can clump together to form a tumour or result in leukaemia:

- **benign tumours** are not cancer. These tumours do not spread to other tissues and do not destroy them unless they push them out of the way or squash them.
- **malignant tumours** (cancer) can grow very quickly, and invade and damage nearby tissues and organs. They may also spread to other parts of the body and form secondary tumours, for example in lymph nodes, lungs, liver and bone.
- **Leukaemia** (see page 101).

Causes

Cancer is thought to have over 200 causes, with most cases due to a combination of factors. Factors known to be linked with cancer include:

- **inherited genes** An increased risk of getting a particular cancer may be inherited from a relative, for example, some breast, ovarian and bowel cancers.
- **smoking** Evidence linking cancer of the lung to cigarette smoking is overwhelming. Smoking can also cause cancer of the mouth, tongue, bladder and other parts of the body.
- **radiation** Damage to cells from radiation can cause leukaemia and cancer of the ovaries, testes and thyroid.
- **sunlight** Too much exposure to ultra violet (UV) radiation in sunlight can cause skin cancer.

Treatment

Early diagnosis is very important because, in most cases, the treatment is less severe and the chances of survival greater. There are three main types of treatment:

- **surgery** to remove the tumour, and sometimes to clear surrounding non-cancerous tissue and lymph nodes to ensure that all cancer cells are removed;
- **chemotherapy** uses medicines to kill cancer cells or stop them spreading;
- **radiotherapy** aims to destroy the cancerous cells with radiation. The dose is carefully controlled to cause as little harm as possible to the surrounding healthy tissue.

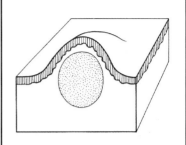

A cyst in the skin
(sebaceous cyst)

Cysts are abnormal pockets of fluid or semi-solid matter which can be mistaken for a cancerous lump. There are many types of cyst and they can occur in different parts of the body including the skin, ovary and breast. Any unusual lumps need to be investigated as a few may be cancerous and need prompt treatment.

2. **a** What is cancer?
   b i How do cells divide,
   ii why does the body need new cells,
   iii what happens when cells multiply in an uncontrolled way?
   c Explain the difference between a benign and a malignant tumour.
   d In two columns, list four factors linked with cancer, and the parts of the body most likely to be affected.
   e Why is early diagnosis of cancer important?
   f Describe three types of treatment.

Routine measurements and observations

It is usual for GPs to offer new patients a routine health check. The purpose is to:

- assess the state of the patient's health;
- offer treatment for any condition discovered;
- offer guidance for any health risk caused by the patient's lifestyle.

Health check

During a new patient's health check:

- the doctor observes the patient's general appearance and mobility, and looks for signs of ill-health;
- the patient's medical and family history is noted and recorded;
- the patient is asked to mention any health concerns they may have;
- routine measurements are taken that form a baseline of the patient's present condition;
- the effectiveness of any present treatment is monitored.

Posture and movements are noted as they can indicate:
- mood (depression, fear);
- loss of mobility (arthritis in hip or knee);
- nervous system problems (stroke, Parkinson's disease).

A stethoscope is used to listen to sounds made inside the body from the:
- heart as it beats;
- lungs during breathing;
- abdomen.

The abdomen is checked for tenderness and swellings, for example:
- enlarged liver, spleen or bladder;
- constipation, appendicitis.

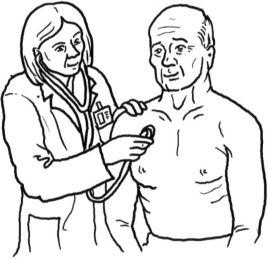

Observations and measurements in a routine health check

Skin colour, texture and body temperature are noted. (➲ pages 191–193.)

The pulse is taken. (➲ page 105.)

Blood pressure is taken. (➲ pages 107 and 137.)

Any shortness of breath or coughing is noted. (➲ pages 111–112.)

A peak flow test may be carried out. (➲ page 112.)

A urine sample is tested (➲ page 119.)

Height, weight and BMI are measured and recorded. (➲ pages 148–9.)

Activity

Produce a booklet to explain how routine measurements and observations can be used as indicators of health or ill-health.

1. a Why do GPs offer new patients a health check?
   b What happens during the health check of a new patient?
   c In a routine health check what aspects of the patient are:
      i   noted/observed by the doctor,
      ii measured, tested or checked in other ways?

Monitoring body systems

Reasons for monitoring

For good health, conditions inside the body need to remain steady and within a certain range (Homeostasis ➲ page 135). Measurements within these limits suggest health: those outside these limits suggest illness.

- **Importance of accuracy** Accurate measurements and not guesses are needed to assess a patient's state of health and they must be recorded correctly.
- **Inaccurate measurements** can occur when not enough time and care are taken to get a correct reading, the correct procedure is not followed or the equipment is faulty.
- **Repeated measurements** are often needed to ensure that the readings are consistent. These need to be taken at the same time of day and under the same conditions.

Observation charts Inpatients in hospitals have a Patient Assessment Folder which contains an Observation Chart to record rates of temperature, pulse, breathing, blood pressure and other readings. The chart is available to doctors, nurses and others who wish to assess the patient's condition and progress.

2. a Why is it important that conditions inside the body keep within a certain range?
 b From the chart when are measurements within normal limits for:
  i temperature,
  ii pulse,
  iii respiration?
 c Why is accuracy important?
 d When may inaccurate measurements occur?
 e Why are repeated measurements taken?
 f What does an observation chart record?

Activity

In your own words, explain how routine measurements and observations can be used as indicators of health and ill-health.

Observation chart of a patient with pneumonia

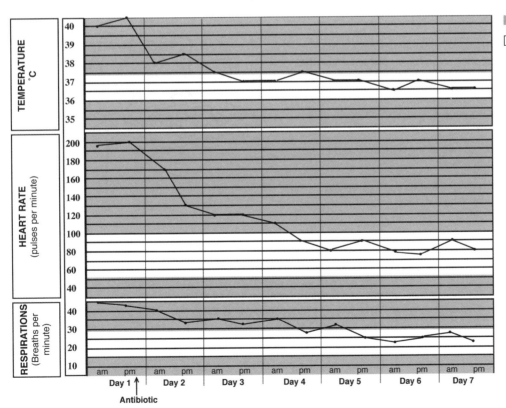

Outside normal limits

Within normal limits

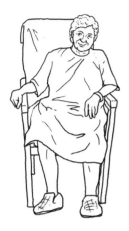

Caring for patients

People who are ill or weak need the same basic care whether they are at home, in hospital, in a nursing home or in residential care. Sitting in a chair is better than spending all day in bed because:

- there is less risk of chest infection and pressure sores;
- it is easier to eat and drink;
- it is less boring as more activities are possible;
- people feel less vulnerable and less dependent.

General care of patients

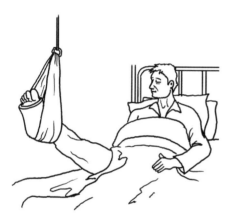

Reduce the risk of deep vein thrombosis (DVT) by encouraging patients to walk if they can, and to do leg and foot exercises regularly if they cannot.

Prevent pressure sores of patients who are unable to move by changing their position regularly, or using aids such as a special mattress or gel pads.

Prevent chest infection by regular deep breathing exercises.

Prevent muscle wasting by encouraging patients to be as active as possible so that they can maintain their mobility and independence.

Attend to toilet needs as soon as possible after the patient's request.

Good ventilation and a **comfortable room temperature**, but no draughts. Older people and babies in particular need warmth to prevent hypothermia.

Provide a suitable diet. Patients need nourishing foods that they are able to eat. Because they often have poor appetites the food needs to look and smell appetising, be served in the right quantities and at the right temperature.

Maintain basic cleanliness as people who are ill or weak have reduced resistance to infection.

Administer the patient's medicines at the right time and in the correct way, and note any side effects.

Prevent boredom by encouraging activities such as talking, reading, doing jigsaws and watching TV.

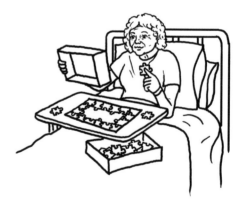

3. a Why are patients not encouraged to spend all day in bed?
   b Describe a suitable diet for patients.
   c Why are ventilation and room temperature important?
   d Why are patients encouraged to be active?
   e What helps to reduce the risk of DVT?
   f Why are activities encouraged?
   g When should carers attend to a patient's toilet needs?
   h When should patients' medicines be given?
   i How can pressure sores be prevented?
   j Which patients need help with basic cleanliness?
   k What helps prevent chest infections?

Health and safety in caring for patients

Hazards and risks

As mentioned on page 50, a **hazard** can be any item, piece of equipment, chemical or biological agent that has the potential to cause harm. **Risk** is any harm that is likely to be caused by a hazard. The hazards and risks shown here are examples of what can occur when caring for patients.

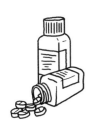
Medicines such as missed doses, the wrong dose, the wrong medicine or an overdose.

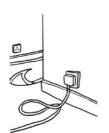
Tripping on steps, upturned carpet or a flex.

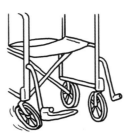
Malfunctioning equipment such as loose wheels or missing foot rests on wheelchairs.

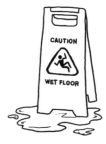
Slipping on wet floors, polished floors, loose mats or spillages.

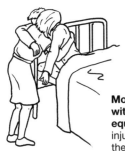
Moving patients without the right equipment can cause injury to the patient or the carer.

Hazards and risks in caring for patients

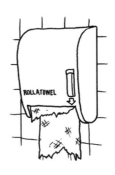
No soap or clean towel for washing and wiping the hands can increase the spread of infection.

Using equipment

Equipment used in health and social care settings should be maintained in good condition, and the staff who use it need to be trained or instructed in its use. For example, trained in the correct:

- use of fire extinguishers and fire blankets;
- use of protective equipment such as plastic aprons and gloves, goggles and masks;
- use of disposable gloves to prevent the spread of infection;
- disposal of soiled and infected linen and other items.

4. **a** What is the difference between a hazard and a risk?
   b Place the hazards and risks above in a table, adding more hazards and risks that you know of.

Hazards	Risks

Activity

Revise 'Health and safety legislation and guidelines' on pages 54–56. Identify the parts of Health and Safety Legislation relevant to patient care.

5. a How can patients find information about their medicines?

  b When a carer is giving medicine:
  i give four points to check,
  ii what should happen afterwards,
  iii what should be noted,
  iv how should the medicine be stored?

  c Name two types of medicine that relieve pain.

  d What type of medicine might be prescribed for:
  i asthma,
  ii indigestion,
  iii diabetes,
  iv hypertension?

Medication

There are many types of medicine each with its own instructions for use and its own Patient Information Leaflet. Remember that medicines should only be given to patients by qualified and registered professionals or under instruction from a qualified and registered professional such as a doctor, nurse or pharmacist.

Points to check when giving medicine to a patient:

- **Always check** that you are giving the right drug to the right patient.
- **Size of dose** – for example, one or two tablets; 5 mg/10 mg; 5 ml/10 ml; two puffs; maximum in a day.
- **Frequency** – for example, one, two, three or four times a day; as necessary.
- **When** – for example, before/after/with meals; on an empty stomach; at bedtime; with water; with other medication - or not.
- **Record** when the medicine has been given with the initials or full name of the person who gave the medicine.
- **Side-effects** – any unwanted symptoms produced by the medicine should be noted.
- **Storage** – medicines must be stored securely, out of the reach of children and in the correct conditions, for example, in a fridge; in a cool place or out of the light.

Examples of medicines, what they do and a precaution

Medicine	Example	Action	Precaution
Acid blockers	ranitidine	reduces stomach acid	see doctor if no better in 2 weeks
Laxatives	senna	relieves constipation	excess causes diarrhoea
Heart tablets	digoxin	strengthens heart beat	narrow dose range
Hypotensives	ramipril	reduces blood pressure	check effect on blood pressure
Diuretics	furosemide	removes excess fluid	check blood pressure not too low
Bronchodilators	salbutamol	opens narrow airways	excess gives tremor & anxiety
Hypnotics	zopiclone	makes drowsy	regular use gives dependence
Antidepressants	doxepin	reduces depression	drowsy, dry mouth, blurred vision
Analgesics	paracetamol	gives pain relief	too much gives liver problems
Antibiotics	amoxicillin	kills bacteria (not viruses)	check that patient is not allergic
Antidiabetic	metformin	reduces blood glucose	healthy diet essential
Iron supplements	ferrous sulphate	treats 'low iron' anaemia	poisonous to children
Anti-inflammatory	ibuprofen	reduces inflammation & pain	stomach irritant – sometimes bleeds

Chapter 6
Human Lifespan Development

This chapter covers:

- The different stages of life and the changes in growth and development that occur.

- The positive and negative influences that affect people at different stages of life.

- The factors that influence self-concept.

- The care needs at different stages of life.

Human growth and development

This section deals with the way that people grow, develop and change throughout life. **Growth** is an increase in size and **development** refers to the increase in abilities (what a person is able to do). Growth and development are most obvious during childhood, but they take place more slowly throughout life. Although life is a continuous process, five main life stages can be identified.

Life stages

Infancy (0–3 years)
Babies and toddlers depend completely on adults for care and protection.

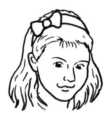

Childhood (4–10 years)
Young children are starting to become independent but still need a great deal of care from adults.

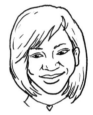

Adolescence (11–18 years)
During this stage children gradually become independent adults.

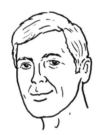

Adulthood (19–65 years)
Adults become parents, grandparents, aunts and uncles. They bring up children and work to support themselves and others.

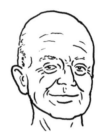

Later adulthood (65+ years)
Generally, people in this age group have fewer responsibilities and more time to enjoy personal interests and hobbies. This life stage can last for 20–30 years or more, with 'old age' now referring to those over 80–85 years.

Aspects of development

The aspects of development include:

- **physical development** – development of the body;
- **intellectual development** – the development of learning, reasoning, problem-solving and speech;
- **social development** – the development of relationships;
- **emotional development** – bonding, independence and self-confidence;
- **personal development** – the way in which a person behaves over time and in different situations.

Activity

Choose someone you know from each of the five life stages. Describe ways in which their life is similar to, or differs from, the generalised description of the life stages given here.

1. **a** What is the difference between growth and development?
   b Describe five life stages.
   c Briefly describe five aspects of development.

Physical development

Conception

Conception occurs when an egg is fertilised. The fertilised egg then starts to develop into a baby and becomes attached to the wall of the uterus by the umbilical cord. An **embryo** is a developing baby during the first seven weeks after conception. It is then called a **fetus** until birth. After 28 weeks development is almost complete and the baby spends the rest of the time in the womb growing larger and stronger.

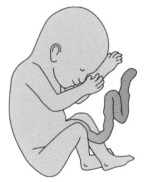

Fetus at 14 weeks.
By now the fetus can swallow, frown, clench the fists and turn the head.

Pregnancy

The genes inherited from the parents control the baby's growth and development but it is also affected by the mother's behaviour. Healthy babies are more likely to be born to:

- mothers who have a nutritious diet that contains folic acid. Folic acid is essential during the first three months of pregnancy to prevent birth defects such as spina bifida.
- mothers who do not smoke, are not overweight, do not regularly drink alcohol, or take drugs or harmful medicines. These substances reach the baby through the placenta and umbilical cord and can adversely affect its development.

Placenta – is attached to the uterus wall and supplies the baby with food and oxygen. It is expelled from the uterus after the baby is born as the afterbirth.

Umbilical cord – links the baby with the placenta. After the birth the cord is cut to release the baby.

Amniotic fluid ('waters') – acts as a cushion and helps to protect the unborn baby from damage.

Uterus (womb) – is made of muscle tissue that expands as the baby grows. During childbirth it contracts and pushes the baby out. After the baby is born, the uterus shrinks back to its usual size.

Cervix (neck of womb) expands during childbirth.

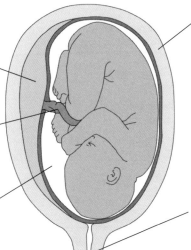

Fetus just before birth

2. **a** When does conception occur?
   b When is a developing baby called:
      i an embryo,   **ii** a fetus?
   c Why is folic acid important in early pregnancy?
   d What substances can adversely affect the development of an unborn baby?
   e What is the purpose of the amniotic fluid?
   f After the baby is born, what happens to the umbilical cord, placenta and uterus?

Growth

Growth is increase in height and weight. Factors that affect the height and weight of an individual are:

- **genetic factors** – the genes inherited from the parents;
- **nutrition** – the overall quality and quantity of food intake;
- **exercise** – the amount taken;
- certain **medical conditions**, for example when the body produces too much or too little thyroid hormone.

Personal Child Health Record (PCHR) Parents are given a Personal Child Health Record in which their child's progress can be recorded. Regular measurements will show if a child's height or weight is outside the normal range. If this occurs, treatment for the child and advice to the parents needs to be given. Children who fail to grow, or grow too much, can suffer socially, emotionally, physically and medically throughout life.

Height

A child's genes determine the maximum height to which the skeleton can grow. Generally, short parents have shorter children than tall parents, and girls are shorter than boys when they have the same biological parents.

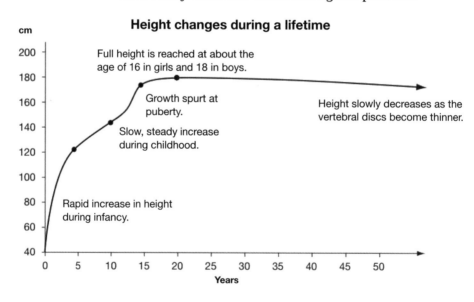

Height changes during a lifetime

Full height is reached at about the age of 16 in girls and 18 in boys.

Growth spurt at puberty.

Slow, steady increase during childhood.

Height slowly decreases as the vertebral discs become thinner.

Rapid increase in height during infancy.

Activity

The **Child Growth Foundation** cares for children who do not grow or grow too much. When was this charity set up and what are its aims?

3. **a** What is growth?
   b What factors affect growth?
   c When and why is it important to be concerned about a child's growth?
   d i What is the purpose of a PCHR,
   ii who enters the information?
   iii why are height and weight recorded,
   iv when and why may treatment be given?
   e Which is the main factor affecting growth in height?
   f Describe height changes that occur during a lifetime.

Weight

Growth in height is accompanied by increase in weight. How much change in weight takes place depends on:

- the genes inherited from the parents;
- how much food is eaten (calories in);
- the amount of exercise taken (calories out).

A healthy weight is one that does not involve too much body fat. This can be assessed by calculating the body mass index and measuring the waist circumference.

Body Mass Index (BMI)

The **BMI** relates a person's weight to their height. It is used as a guide to a healthy weight. **BMI charts** show the ideal weight for most men and women. But they are not intended for pregnant or breast-feeding women, weight-trainers, athletes or people with a long-term health condition.

BMI for children is calculated in the same way as for adults but the results are interpreted using special charts for children. These charts are age- and sex-related because the amount of body fat differs between boys and girls, and changes with age.

Waist circumference

This is a good indicator of abdominal fat and a predictor of the risk for developing diseases associated with obesity. The measurement is taken by placing a tape measure around the waist. In adults, a measurement of over 100 cm (40 inches) in men and over 90 cm (35 inches) in women indicates an increased health risk.

Diseases associated with obesity

People who are overweight are more likely to have health problems due to:

- high blood pressure (hypertension), which is a major risk for heart disease and stroke;
- high cholesterol levels;
- diabetes.

The risk of developing these diseases is further increased by:

- a family history of the conditions named above;
- physical inactivity;
- cigarette smoking.

Calculating BMI

BMI is calculated by dividing the body's weight in kilograms by height in metres squared:

$$\frac{\text{weight in kg}}{\text{height} \times \text{height in m}}$$

Example

When weight is 63 kilograms (kg) and height is 1.6 metres (m), then:

$$\frac{63}{1.6 \times 1.6}$$

$$= \frac{63}{2.56}$$

$$= 24.6 \text{ BMI}$$

Adults BMI Chart

Underweight	BMI less than 18.5
Ideal	BMI 18.5–24.9
Overweight	BMI 25–29.9
Obese	BMI 30–39.9
Very obese	BMI greater than 40

---

4. **a** What two actions affect weight?
   b What is a healthy weight?
   c **i** What is BMI,
   ii what does it indicate,
   iii why is it used?
   d Who are BMI charts not intended for?
   e **i** Describe how to calculate BMI,
   ii what does BMI 24.6 indicate?
   f Why are BMI charts for adults not used for children?
   g When does waist circumference indicate being overweight?
   h **i** Which diseases are linked with being overweight,
   ii when is the risk increased?

Activity

Calculate your BMI and measure your waist circumference. What do they indicate about your weight?

Infancy (0-3 years)

Physical development

During the first few years of life, infants grow and develop rapidly from being a helpless baby to an independent child.

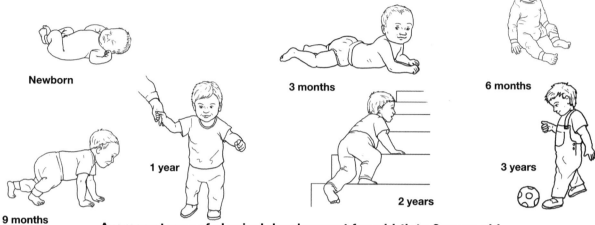

Average stages of physical development from birth to 3 years old

Age stage	Movements	Hands	Eyes	Voice
Newborn	Kicks, stretches, moves arms and turns head.	Hands are usually closed.	Aware of light and movement but very short-sighted.	Cries when hungry, lonely or in pain.
3 months	Lifts head when lying face downwards.	Hands are usually open.	Very interested in things nearby, especially faces.	Gurgles, babbles and holds 'conversations' with people.
6 months	Sits with support.	Uses hands to grasp toys.	Eyes work together and are rarely crossed.	Makes a variety of sounds.
9 months	Tries to crawl.	Uses hands to drop things on floor.	Can see further.	Makes sounds 'dad-dad', 'mum-mum' and 'bab-bab'.
1 year	Begins to walk.	Points to things.	Recognises people at a distance.	Says a few words with meaning such as 'bye-bye'.
2 years	Climbs up the stairs.	Holds a pencil and scribbles.	Can see as far as an adult can see.	Makes simple sentences.
3 years	Kicks a ball.	Uses a spoon without spilling.	Begins to recognise colours.	Talks continuously.

Activity

Find a picture of a child at each of the seven age stages. Arrange them in order then add labels to indicate what most children of that age are able to do in movement, use of the hands, eyes and voice.

Intellectual development

From birth onwards, everything a child does gives them a chance for learning, and much of this learning takes place through play. Play enables young children to make sense of their world and helps with the development of problem-solving.

Emotional development

Emotional development is learning to recognise emotions (feelings) and to control them. Babies come into the world with strong feelings. They cry when they are feeling hungry, tired, uncomfortable or lonely. When a baby is held close to another person, it gets feelings of comfort and security.

Providing loving care and attention allows **bonds of attachment** (strong feelings of affection) to form between parents and child. The child will then feel secure and develop a positive view of itself, with the self-confidence to explore the world it lives in and the ability to bounce back from disappointments. A sense of security enables a child to develop good relationships with others, an ability which continues into adult life.

Social development

This is the process of learning the skills that enable individuals to live easily with other people. New babies are social beings right from the start and have an inborn need for the company of other people. They soon come to recognise their mother or main carer. When a few weeks old, they smile at people and by 9 months they can recognise strangers. At the age of about 2 years they like to play near other children and by 3 years they want to play with them.

Learning the rules By 1 year old most children have begun to understand the meaning of 'NO' and they gradually come to realise that parents are pleased by some things they do and not by others. When children are old enough to understand what is wanted of them, they benefit from rules that are reasonable and consistent. This helps them learn to behave in a way acceptable to other people.

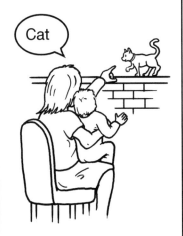

How babies learn to talk
They learn from adults by copying the sounds and what they mean. For example . . .

Cat

. . . when an adult points to a cat and says 'cat' the baby copies the sound and says 'cat'. By repeating sounds, the baby learns what the sounds mean. A vocabulary is gradually built up, and words linked together to form sentences.

4. **a** Why is play important for young children?
   b How do babies learn to talk?
   c How do babies show their feelings?
   d i What is a bond of attachment,
   ii how does it affect the child's feelings,
   iii how can it affect relationships?
   e What is social development?
   f Describe social development from birth to 3 years.
   g At what age do children begin to learn about rules?
   h What rules benefit a child, and why?

Activity

Find some pictures of children at the different stages of social development. Place them in sequence and add captions.

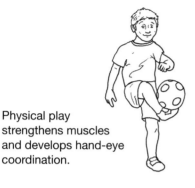

Physical play
strengthens muscles
and develops hand-eye
coordination.

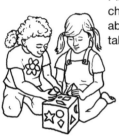

Playing with other
children teaches
about sharing and
taking turns.

Playing with toys enables
children to discover about size,
shape, gravity, weight, rigidity,
flexibility and breaking.

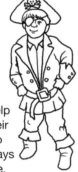

Pretend games help
children to use their
imagination and to
understand the ways
that others behave.

Childhood (4-10 years)

Humans have a very long childhood and this gives time for learning the skills needed for adult life:

- physical skills such as use of the fingers (fine motor skills) and walking (a gross motor skill);
- skilled use of language;
- literacy skills – to read and to write clearly;
- numeracy skills – to use numbers;
- social skills;
- problem-solving and decision-making.

Play

It is natural for children to want to play. Play is an important part of children's lives because while they are playing they are learning about themselves, other people and their environment. When they draw, make or build something and are praised for their achievements it helps to build positive self-esteem.

Physical development

There is little difference in average size between boys and girls and, at this age, they develop at a similar rate. Boys tend to be more active and enjoy energetic and physically aggressive games. Girls tend to prefer less energetic activities and friendships are very important.

Intellectual development

The brain grows quickly during childhood and by the age of six it has already reached 90% of the adult weight. During this stage, children learn rapidly about the world around them. Young children have vivid imaginations and enjoy playing pretend games. They have difficulty distinguishing fantasy from reality, but gradually they become able to reason, solve problems, understand other people's points of view, and to compromise with them.

Learning to read Even before 18 months of age, children can listen to and understand a story being read to them. When hearing stories is a source of pleasure, children will be more eager to learn to read for themselves. A child's educational chances and opportunities in life are increased by being able to read and write easily.

Activity

Describe some play activities that require:
i   literacy skills,
ii numeracy skills.

5. a Why is a long childhood an advantage to humans?
   b i   Why do children play,
     ii what benefits of play are shown in the pictures above,
     iii when can play help build self-esteem,
     iv do boys and girls play differently?
   c How does the brain develop during childhood?
   d What is the benefit of reading stories to children?

Emotional development

Children's feelings can affect development in many ways, and of special importance are the feelings of security and insecurity.

- **Secure children feel safe** – safe from being hurt and from being lonely, unhappy, rejected and afraid. They know that there is always someone who cares and a place where they belong. Secure children are more likely to settle well into school, work cooperatively, confidently and independently and to behave appropriately.
- **Insecure children feel unloved and unwanted**. This can make them timid and withdrawn or indulge in bad behaviour in order to attract attention. They then soon learn that 'bad' behaviour makes people notice them, while to be 'good' often results in being ignored.

Social development

Social development (**socialisation**) is learning to live easily with other people. Children and adults are happier when they have the social skills that enable them to get on well with others.

Social skills are those used to interact with other people:
- the ability to talk easily with other people;
- knowing how to share, take turns and accept rules;
- respect for other people and their property;
- having standards of cleanliness acceptable to others;
- eating in a manner that does not offend others;
- thanking people when something is done for them;
- apologising when they are in the wrong;
- tolerance of other people's differing opinions, beliefs and behaviour.

Discipline

Discipline that is both reasonable and consistent helps to teach children about the rules and boundaries of acceptable behaviour.

Lack of discipline is harmful when it results in children who are:

- **insecure** – because no limits are placed on their behaviour;
- **disobedient and uncooperative** – in order to get attention;
- **rude** – they do not consider other people's feelings;
- **accident-prone** – they are not taught to be aware of danger.

Too much discipline is also harmful because it:

- demands too much of a child - too much obedience or tidiness;
- can result in a child who is shy, timid and lacking in self-esteem.

6. a What makes children feel secure?
   b How do insecure children feel?
   c Compare the likely behaviour of children who feel secure with those who feel insecure.
   d What are social skills?
   e When is discipline for children:
      i helpful,
      ii harmful?

Adolescence

Adolescence is the stage of transition from child to adult. It covers several years and, during this time, changes occur in all aspects of development.

Physical development

As growth continues, the greater muscle development in males makes them stronger than females, whereas females tend to be lighter and more supple than males.

Adolescence begins with **puberty** – the stage during which the sex organs grow and become able to function. It usually starts sometime between the ages of 10-15 years with the time taken to complete this stage varying widely among normal children. Puberty is controlled by hormones – testosterone in males and oestrogen and progesterone in females. During puberty and a year or two afterwards, the child has to adjust to an altered system of hormones, a changing body shape, and the effects that the hormones have on the emotions and on sexual identity.

7. **a** Explain the difference between adolescence and puberty.
   b What are the effects of muscle development?
   c i When does puberty usually start,
   ii what is it controlled by?
   d Describe four changes that a child has to adjust to during puberty?

Physical changes that take place at puberty

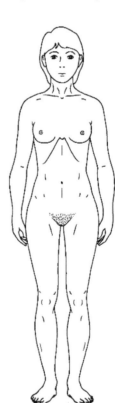

Male characteristics

Skin becomes oily and may cause acne.

Beard grows.

Voice breaks.

Shoulders broaden.

Hair grows in armpits and may grow on chest.

Muscles develop.

Pubic hair grows.

Penis grows.

Testes grow and start to produce sperm.

Female characteristics

Skin becomes oily and may cause acne.

Breasts grow.

Hair grows in armpits.

Hips broaden.

Pubic hair grows.

Ovaries grow and start to produce eggs.

Uterus enlarges and periods (menstruation) begins.

Vagina enlarges.

Activity

Draw an outline of an adolescent male. Add labels of the physical changes that take place at puberty. Repeat using an outline of an adolescent female.

Intellectual development

Adolescence is a time when facts are easily absorbed and education is a preparation for adult life. Teenagers have the ability to plan ahead and solve problems but do not yet have the experience to reason in an adult way.

Emotional development

During adolescence children move from dependence on their parents to independence. Those with more self-confidence and a supportive family find it easier to make the transition. Those lacking self-esteem or who feel isolated or rejected by their family are more likely to associate with others with similar problems, and engage in risky antisocial behaviours in order to fit in with the group.

Social development

As children become adolescents they enter a new phase in their relationships with others. Although parents continue to be important, teenagers want to spend more time with people of their own age (their **peer group**) and without adult supervision. The influence of their peers is very important in a teenager's life and can outweigh their parents' opinions. But they need to learn how to cope with disagreements and to compromise with an often unsympathetic world of adults.

Peer pressure is the pressure to be like everyone else in the peer group. It is often very important for teenagers to be like their friends in wearing the same clothes, listening to a particular type of music, and so on. Pressure from the group can be very influential and teenagers learn a lot from their peers:

- **positive peer pressure** can help young people to form the values and attitudes that will motivate them to succeed;
- **negative peer pressure** can impair good judgement and fuel dangerous risk-taking behaviour, drawing a teenager away from the family and into harmful activities.

Sexual activity During adolescence adolescents become sexually active. They need to be aware that unprotected sex can result in an unwanted pregnancy and sexually-transmitted diseases. These can result in emotional problems such as unhappiness, guilt and quarrels.

8. **a** Describe the teenagers' stage of intellectual development.
   b Which two factors make it easier to learn?
   c i Describe the transition in emotional development,
   ii who is likely to find it easier?
   iii who is likely to find it harder?
   d Describe the changing relationship between teenagers and parents.
   e i What is peer pressure,
   ii how does positive and negative peer pressure differ?
   f Give two possible results of unprotected sex.

Activity

Take part in a discussion on:
a In what ways do teenagers think differently from adults?
b Is peer pressure a good thing or a bad thing?

Adulthood

Adults usually move away from the family home and select a partner to share their life with. They make their own decisions and are responsible for their own health. They also have the pressures of earning a living and holding down a job. This age group is responsible for the care of children and the older members of the family.

Physical development

After puberty, growth in height stops, but muscles continue to build, depending on how much they are used. Peak performance in highly active sports is in the late teens to early thirties. After that, strength and speed gradually decline but regular exercise at any age helps to maintain physical fitness. 'Middle-aged spread' occurs when adults have become much less active and continue to eat the same amount of food as before.

Intellectual development

Adults develop a greater understanding of themselves and their abilities and limitations. They become more able to take a long-term view and show less impulsive behaviour. Although brain development is complete, adults can continue to gain new skills, hobbies, interests and jobs.

Emotional development

Most adults feel secure and ready for stable relationships and commitments for the future.

Social development

Peer group relationships dwindle and are replaced by a wider circle of friendships that include work colleagues and people with similar interests.

Producing children

Women are most fertile in their late teens and early twenties, and conceive children more easily. The risk of miscarriage, complications at birth and the birth of a child with disabilities increases with age. After the menopause at about the age of 50, the ovaries stop producing eggs and women cease to be fertile.

Fertility in men decreases as they become older and produce fewer sperm. **Impotence** (failure to maintain an erection) can occur at any age but occurs more commonly in older men.

Infertility (sterility) is the inability to conceive. There are many reasons for this, and couples who want children can obtain advice from GPs and Family Planning clinics.

9. **a** List seven aspects of adult life.
   b Describe the stage reached by adults in:
      i intellectual development,
      ii emotional development,
      iii social development.
   c i What happens to the muscles of adults,
      ii when is peak performance reached,
      iii what helps to maintain physical fitness,
      iv why does middle-aged spread develop?
   d i At what age do women produce children more easily,
      ii what increases with age,
      iii when do they become infertile?
   e Do men remain fertile?
   f What is impotence?
   g i What is infertility,
      ii where can advice be obtained?

Activity

Describe the key aspects of physical, intellectual, emotional and social development through the life stages from infancy to adulthood.

Parenthood

Parenting is carried out by adults (usually the parents) who provide care for children. Bringing up children is a long-term job and the way in which a child is brought up will have an effect for the rest of the child's life. Parents cannot be perfect but when they are loving and caring and take an interest in their children's development, the children are less vulnerable to stress, have better social skills and more successful relationships.

Parenting young children

When children are young, their development is helped when their parents:

- play with them – this helps to develop both mind and body;
- talk to them – this teaches a child how to speak;
- answers their questions – this increases vocabulary and knowledge;
- read to them – this helps in the process of learning to read and listen;
- are involved in their education – this is likely to result in children who enjoy school, get better academic results and have fewer problems with their behaviour.

Activity

Role play 'Parents of teenagers' based on the six items in the list on this page. (➲ Role play, page 244.)

Parents of teenagers

It is natural for parents to want to protect their children. It is also essential for teenagers to learn to be responsible adults. This is helped when parents:

- keep the lines of communication open between them and their teenage children;
- accept that their teenagers are young adults and no longer dependent children;
- offer them choices rather than telling them what to do;
- give them opportunities to make their own decisions and to learn by their mistakes;
- respect their need for privacy and independence;
- continue to offer guidance and support.

Parenting classes

These are intended for parents who feel that they need advice or those who are having problems with their children's behaviour. These classes are based on **positive parenting**. This includes showing affection and respect for their child, praising the behaviour they want, and ignoring (when possible) naughty behaviour. Evidence shows that children with parents who use such skills are far less likely to have behaviour problems.

10. **a** List six ways that parents can help teenagers become responsible adults.
   b Which parents are parenting classes intended for?
   c What is meant by positive parenting?
   d Complete the table below.

Parenting young children

Action by parents	Benefit to children
Playing with children	

Ageing

Ageing is a natural process and results in gradual changes to various parts of the body that prevent them from functioning as efficiently as they once did. The different parts of the body age at different rates, for example:

- the skin begins to lose its elasticity in early adult life;
- eyesight and hearing become less efficient from the mid-forties;
- the number of brain cells decreases throughout life – although there are many millions of brain cells left, it becomes more difficult to remember recent events than it is to recall those that happened many years ago;
- arteries begin to clog up from childhood onwards, a process that is encouraged by lack of exercise, over-eating and smoking; clogged arteries can be the cause of heart attacks and stroke.

The rate at which people age depends on:

- inherited genes;
- attitude to life;
- state of health;
- money – on average, rich people live longer than poor people and age more slowly.

Activity

Explain how growth and development at each life stage can be influenced positively and negatively. (➲ pages 148-158.)

Height is lost because the discs in the backbone become thinner.

Posture may become bent due to habit or a health problem.

Joints stiffen due to 'wear and tear', **falls** are more common.

Bones break more easily due to loss of calcium and protein.

Muscles become weaker.

Recall of recent events may be more difficult.

Reaction times are slower.

Eyesight may be impaired as the lens loses its elasticity and if cataracts develop.

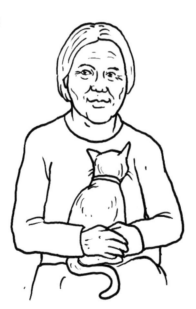

Keeping warm is more difficult due to less movement and less awareness of being cold.

Hearing becomes less acute, especially the high notes.

Sense of smell decreases, making it more difficult to detect escaping gas, bad food and other smells.

Hair turns grey, becomes thinner and may be lost.

Wrinkles develop as skin becomes less elastic.

Skin becomes thinner resulting in easier bruising.

Movements become slower due to stiffer joints and weaker muscles.

Changes that happen as you grow older

11. **a i** What is ageing,   **ii** why do people age at different rates?
    b As people grow older, what happens to their:
       i brain cells,   **ii** arteries,   **iii** eyesight and hearing?
    c What changes happen to the:
       i ability to keep warm (1 answer),   **ii** recall (1 answer),   **iii** sense organs (3 answers),
       iv appearance (5 answers),   **v** muscles, bones and movement (6 answers).

Why 'use it or lose it'?

If the body and brain are not used, the ability to use them will decline. To help delay the effects of ageing people can:

- take regular exercise because muscles that are not used weaken;
- avoid becoming overweight because it puts strain on the heart and joints, and makes diabetes and heart disease more likely;
- keep mentally active because a brain that is not used deteriorates;
- keep interested in other people and events because it helps to prevent boredom and loneliness;
- have a well-balanced diet to keep healthy;
- take care of the feet because painful feet makes walking difficult and reduces mobility.

The final stages of life

As people grow older, various systems in the body become less efficient and more subject to disease. The main causes of death in the UK are diseases related to ageing – heart disease, stroke and cancer. Whatever the cause, death occurs when the heart stops beating, the brain stops working and breathing stops.

Individuals vary in the way they approach death. Some may want the support of their family and friends; others may wish to die alone. Some may be afraid of dying and prefer not to think about it whereas some very old people or those who are very ill may feel that it is time to let go of life. Traditions and beliefs associated with death are a part of human culture and central to many religions. They are therefore important to many people and need to be observed according to the beliefs and wishes of the dying person.

12. a What happens to the body and brain when not used?

b Describe six ways to help delay the effect of ageing.

c What are the main causes of death in the UK?

d How do individuals vary in the way they approach death?

e Why are the traditions and beliefs associated with death important?

Activity

Cruse Bereavement Care is a voluntary organisation. Find out why it exists, what services it offers and where your nearest branch is. Present your findings as a leaflet designed for older people and their relatives.

Factors that influence personal development

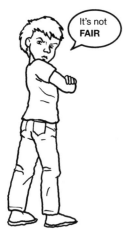

Young children have a strong sense of what is right and what is wrong, and they object strongly to situations that they think are unjust. If they are given an explanation, it may help to soothe their feelings and teach them how to cope with what they see as injustice.

1. a i What is socialisation,
  ii Why is it a continuing process?
  b What part do families play in primary socialisation?
  c i What is secondary socialisation,
  ii when does it begin,
  iii who are children influenced by?
  d i what is moral development,
  ii what is it influenced by?
  e What is a conscience?
  f What are moral values?
  g What may encourage the development of poor moral values?

Activity

Discuss your own moral values with other students. Where did your moral values come from and how did you learn them? Are your values the same as other students? If not, why do you think this is?

Factors that influence an individual's personal development are:

- interactions with other people;
- economic circumstances;
- life's events.

These factors may have positive effects on the individual that are helpful to development or negative effects that are unhelpful.

Socialisation

Socialisation (social development) is learning to become part of a social group. It is a continuing process throughout life as individuals adapt to different social groups, for example pre-school groups, primary school, secondary school, the workplace and retirement.

- **Primary socialisation** begins within the family. Families have beliefs about the right way to behave and what attitudes, customs and values are considered normal. These play an important part in forming young children's values, attitudes and beliefs, many of which may remain for life.
- **Secondary socialisation** is learning to become part of a wider group. It begins when young children become aware of people outside the home and how they behave. Children are also influenced by friends at school and the attitudes of their peer group, which may have different values, attitudes and beliefs to the family.

Moral development

Moral development is learning to know the difference between right and wrong. It is part of the socialisation process and is influenced by:

- guidance and example from parents and teachers;
- the behaviour of friends, the peer group and other people in the locality;
- people in the media who, though never met, can become role models.

As a result of moral development, an individual acquires a **conscience**, which is an internal set of moral values that each person learns to live by. **Moral values** are those shared by a social group and may include the values of caring for each other, of honesty and of putting the interests of the community before one's own. Watching others behave in an antisocial way can encourage the development of poor moral values.

Social behaviour

Social behaviour is the way that a person relates to other people. Children learn how to behave towards others by:

- **observation** – watching the way family members, adults, their peers and people in the media behave;
- **imitation** – copying the behaviour of other people;
- **rewards** – rewarding good behaviour by giving praise and by showing an interest in a child's activities – children who get attention only when behaving badly will continue to behave badly in order to be noticed.

Pro-social behaviour

Pro-social behaviour involves sharing, helping and caring. A willingness to be cooperative and helpful towards other people is learned more quickly when children:

- discuss behaviour, good or bad, with their parents and teachers;
- when parents and teachers are role models who show such behaviour themselves;
- are rewarded by praise and affection when behaving well, and ignored (when possible) when they are difficult.

Anti-social behaviour

Anti-social behaviour is harmful or annoying to others and includes:

- mental abuse from endless teasing and bullying;
- physical abuse, for example pushing, hitting, biting, spitting;
- damaging and stealing property;
- deliberate disruption of other people's activities.

Anti-social behaviour in children can develop when they:

- imitate the anti-social behaviour of parents, carers, teachers or peers;
- get into the habit of stealing anything they want such as sweets, money or mobile phones;
- are rewarded or praised for anti-social behaviour.

Punishment

Punishments such as smacking and shouting may have only a short-term effect. The long-term use of physical punishment for children can make them timid and withdrawn or aggressive towards others.

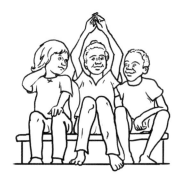

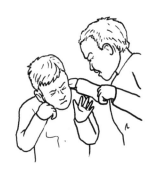

2. a What is social behaviour?
   b How do children learn to behave towards other people?
   c What is pro-social behaviour?
   d What helps children to learn to behave in a pro-social way?
   e Describe anti-social behaviour.
   f What encourages anti-social behaviour in children?

Activities

1. Give examples of anti-social behaviour and your reaction to it.
2. Is smacking children illegal? Find out the current situation in England and Wales. Is it different in Scotland and in Northern Ireland? (⊃ page 245 Media search.) What are your own views on smacking children?

Socio-economic factors

Socio-economic factors are those related to social (people-related) and economic (money-related; financial) matters such as income, housing, education and life-style activities.

Income and expenditure

Income is money received by individuals or households either as payment for work or from welfare benefits, pensions, interest on savings and dividends from stocks and shares.

Expenditure is money that is spent. Money is used for housing, food, clothing, heating, transport, possessions and leisure activities.

Debt People get into debt when expenditure exceeds income and there is not enough money to pay the bills, for example the mortgage and credit cards. Worrying about debt can result in:

- anxiety and depression with disturbed sleep and moody irritable behaviour and other stress-related ill-health (➲ page 40);
- a break down in relationships.

Effects of a low income (➲ page 33)

Poverty is usually defined as a household that lives on an income that is less than 60% of the average household income in the country where they live (after housing costs have been removed). There is then not enough money to do the things that other people consider normal or essential. Poverty therefore reduces the opportunities of having:

- a secure home;
- good health;
- a clean environment;
- a balanced diet;
- a decent education;
- a choice of jobs;
- a choice of leisure activities;
- holidays and travel;
- a long retirement.

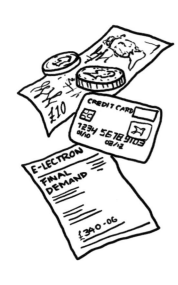

Activities

1. Make a list of the items in your life that you consider essential. Describe how you would feel if there was no money to pay for them?

2. Give a talk for at least four minutes on the impact that debt can have on mental health. Use the internet to carry out some research on this topic. Use your research results in your talk. (➲ page 242 Giving a talk.)

3. a i What are socio-economic factors?
     ii Give three examples.
   b i Where does income come from,
     ii what is an income needed for?
   c i When do people get into debt,
     ii what may be the effects of worry?
   d How is poverty defined?
   e In what ways does poverty reduce life's opportunities?

The influence of socio-economic factors

Factors	Positive influences on development	Negative influences on development
Housing	Housing which feels comfortable and safe, with enough space for everyone and a secure water and energy supply.	Uncomfortable house and worries about safety, cold, damp, unfriendly neighbours and a threatening neighbourhood.
Environment	Clean, healthy and safe.	Overcrowded, unsafe and unhealthy surroundings.
Family	Supportive, non-judgemental.	Adverse destructive criticism, indifference or abuse.
Friends	Friends interested in your well-being and who can be depended on for support.	Unreliable friends, drug addicts and criminals.
Peer pressure	Independent decisions respected.	Pressure and threats to copy others.
Media	Items with good information.	Items which misrepresent information.
Culture	Proud of the culture to which you belong and tolerant towards the culture of others.	Ashamed of your cultural background and intolerant of other cultures.
Gender	Happy with your gender.	Unhappy with your gender.
Discrimination	People's differences are valued.	Unfair discrimination.
Education	Better use made of opportunities.	Poor opportunities, or have not taken advantage of those available.
Access to services	Easy when you need them.	Difficult or impossible.

Activity

For each of the factors above, give your own example of a positive influence and a negative influence on development. Record your answers in a chart.

Social and economic influences on development

Factor	Positive influence	Negative influence
Housing		

Life events

Life events are the major changes that take place during life. They can be predictable or unpredictable.

- **Predictable events** happen to everyone as they pass through the different stages of life. It is often possible to plan ahead for them and to get used to the idea of the changes that will take place.
- **Unpredictable events** are the unexpected ones. Some are stressful because they are unexpected and can then cause medium or long-term unhappiness. But some are desirable and exciting partly because they are unexpected.

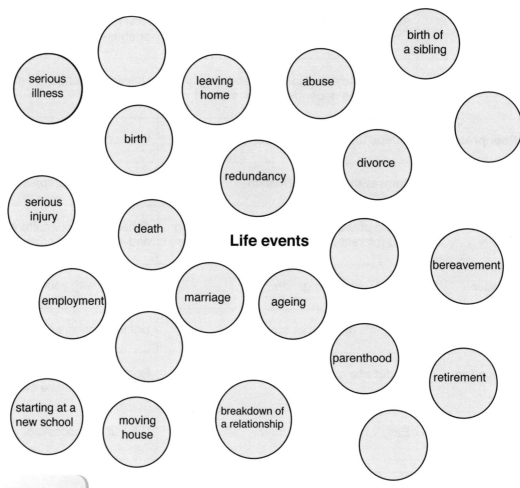

4. a From the life events named above, choose:
   i two that are predictable,
   ii six that happen to most people,
   iii four that are unpredictable.
   b Suggest five other life events for the empty circles.

Activities

1. Choose five of the life events and, for each, give a positive example and a negative example of how that event can affect the lives of individuals. Present your results in a table. Discuss your answers with other students.
2. Explain how life events can affect the development and care needs of individuals.

Adapting to change

Many changes occur during a lifetime - growing up, growing older, relationships, friendships, education, jobs, health, death. How a person copes with change depends on the circumstances:

- the individual's self-confidence, personality and general outlook on life;
- how the event is handled;
- if harm is involved;
- support from family and friends;
- whether the changes are short-term, medium-term or long-term.

Positive effects of change

Sometimes changes have a positive effect and the individual feels good about them, for example when:

- passing an exam or getting a better job;
- moving to a new area results in a happier home;
- retirement allows time for new and interesting challenges.

Changes that are stressful

Changes have a negative effect and are stressful when:

- becoming unemployed makes for uncertainty about the future;
- bereavement creates a sense of loss about the way things used to be;
- retirement when it results in loss of a sense of purpose, of income and of status;
- ill-health or injury destroys lifestyle and ambition.

Negative ⇨ positive effects

Sometimes negative changes can bring about positive results. For example, if a person injured themselves due to their own antisocial behaviour, and the shock caused that person's behaviour to change for the better, the outcome could be regarded as positive.

5. a What circumstances affect a person's ability to cope with change?
b Give examples of the:
  i positive effects of change,
  ii negative effects of change.
c Give an example of a negative change that can have a positive effect.

Activity

Choose a biography or autobiography written about someone you are interested in. From the account of that person's life, note events that:
i were predictable;
ii were unpredictable;
iii had a positive effect;
iv had a negative effect;
v had a short-term, medium-term or long-term effect;
vi were negative, then turned out to have a positive effect.

Self-concept

Do I look good in this?

I enjoy my job and the people I work with.

I never do anything right.

I know that I'm better than they are.

Self-concept is 'who you think you are' and is a combination of self-image and self-esteem.

Self-image is your internal picture of yourself – what you look like and how you behave. It develops in response to what others say to you, how they describe you and how they behave towards you.

Self-esteem is how you value yourself as a person.

- **Positive self-esteem** means that a person feels generally happy about who they are and that they are valued by others.
- **Low (negative) self-esteem** applies to people who have a low opinion of themselves. This can come from the lack of appreciation or constant criticism by other people which makes a person feel worthless. Low self-esteem can be the cause of depression and anxiety.
- **High (inflated) self-esteem** applies to people who rate themselves higher than they are rated by others, and they can seem arrogant and self-centred.

Factors that influence self-concept

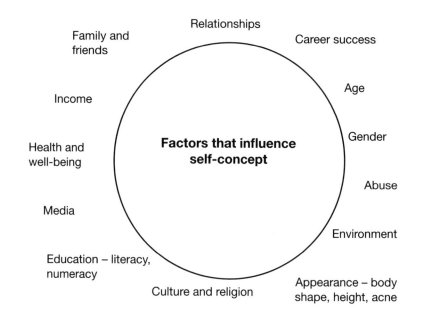

1. a i What is self-concept,
   ii What factors influence self-concept?
   b What is the difference between self-image and self-esteem?
   c How does self-image develop?
   d What is the effect of positive self-esteem?
   e Explain the difference between low and high self-esteem.
   f From the speech bubbles above, choose one that illustrates:
   i self-image,
   ii positive self-esteem,
   iii low self-esteem,
   iv high self-esteem.

Activity

Describe your own self-image. What do you think you look like and how would you describe your behaviour? How do you think others regard you and how does their reaction to you affect your self-concept?

Relationships

Relationships are personal links with other people. There are different types:

- **family relationships** are the first to be formed and affect the development of self-concept by the children. Friendly comments about a child's appearance and behaviour help to produce a positive self-image in the child. Parents who make their children feel special and praise their achievements help to build their self-esteem. Children who are neglected or constantly criticised, develop a poor self-image and feel worthless and resentful.
- **social relationships** with friends and peers provide opportunities for giving and receiving mutual support.
- **working relationships** take place within education and employment.
- **sexual relationships** involving love and care in a partnership are a deeply satisfying experience.
- **caring relationships** are links between those being cared for and their professional or informal carers.

Factors that increase self-concept	Factors that can result in low self-concept
Infancy	**Infancy**
Secure bond of attachment with parents or carers	Failure to make secure bonds of attachment
A loving home	Adults show little interest in the child
Many opportunities to learn	Feelings of being neglected
Childhood	**Childhood**
A loving home that makes the child feel special	A stressful home
Happy at school and praised for achievement	Lack of confidence in abilities
Friends to play with	Difficulty in making friends
Adolescence	**Adolescence**
Supportive family	Conflict with parents and family
Able to develop interests outside the family	Reluctance to be a responsible adult
Sharing a common culture with a group of friends	Few friends and feeling rejected by the peer group
Adulthood	**Adulthood**
Secure sexual relationships	Unsuccessful sexual relationships
Good relationships at work	Unvalued by colleagues at work
Supportive network of family and friends	Little support from the family
Old age	**Old age**
A network of family and friends for support	Few friends and little support
Being valued	Loneliness
Opportunities for involvement with other people	Isolation

Activity

Thinking about your own life:
i   what relationships do you have with other people,
ii which conditions have increased, or lowered, your self-concept?

Age

As individuals grow up and grow older, their self-concept changes. For example, a girl's self-image will change as she moves from her teens to her twenties. It will also change if she becomes a mother and, again, if she becomes a grandmother. The self-concept of older people depends partly on how the society in which they live regards old age – in a negative way or as something to be valued and respected.

Appearance

About the age of ten, children start to analyse the ways in which they are like and unlike others – their self-image. They become conscious of what they wear and how they look. Self-esteem, particularly in young people, may be lowered when they feel unhappy with their body shape or their appearance, or they are not dressed like their peers. It is also lowered if they are 'picked on' for being unusual in some way such as being too fat, disfigured, having a disability, or just too different from the accepted average – short, tall or they have red hair.

Gender

Children become aware of being a boy or a girl early in life. How gender affects their self-esteem can be influenced by whether their parents are happy with their child or would have preferred one of the opposite gender. A girl's self-esteem can be damaged if she is unable to achieve what she wants to do because she is not male. Males may suffer from low self-esteem if they do not fit into their gender stereotype. For example, boys who are skinny or not sporty may feel that they are not masculine enough. Children with homosexual feelings may suffer low-esteem because they cannot be open about their feelings.

Culture

Fulfilling the expectations of a particular cultural or ethnic group enhances self-esteem; feeling inadequate lowers self-esteem. For example, if it is the culture for young males to have a tough image, those that do will feel superior to those who don't. Those who go against the expectations of their social group, for example absentee fathers and ex-prisoners, may have low self-esteem.

2. **a** What does self-concept in older people partly depend on?
   b When do children become:
      i aware of their self-image,
      ii aware of their gender?
   c Give three examples of how gender can affect self-esteem.
   d How may culture affect a person's self-esteem?

Religion

Religion can affect self-concept. Many religions give their followers a sense of self-worth. However, people who grow up as part of a religious family and then change or reject their religion may have a low self-concept because they feel like an outcast and resent the pressure to conform.

Health and well-being

Self-concept is affected by a person's state of health. Knowing that you look fit improves self-image, and feeling fit improves self-esteem.

Income

Self-concept can be influenced by the family's income. Having enough money gives security, whereas being short of money is stressful and reduces opportunities.

Education

Self-esteem can be influenced by educational achievements, or the lack of them. Low achievement can produce feelings of failure, depression and reduced opportunities.

Media

The media includes television, radio, newspapers, magazines and mass advertisements. These strongly influence our concepts of self-image. 'Adverts' often associate happiness with material possessions and sexual success – you would be happy if you owned the latest gadget or a new car or expensive cosmetics, and unhappy if you don't.

Environment

The area where people live can affect self-concept. Living in high crime areas can cause anxiety about the well-being and safety of the family. When the children do not have secure places to play off the streets, or where they can be entertained, occupied and kept busy, they may have little pride in where they live and low self-concept.

3. a How may self-concept be increased by:
   i religion,
   ii health and well-being,
   iii income,
   iv education?
   b How may low self-concept result from:
   i religion,
   ii income,
   iii education,
   iv the media,
   v the environment?

Activity

Describe how five different factors can influence the development of an individual's self-concept.

Care needs

People in need of care are the young, the old and those who are sick, disabled and distressed. The physical, social, emotional and intellectual needs of individuals are dealt with in Chapter 2. Here we are dealing with service users' care needs.

There are different types of care, for example:

- medical and nursing care provided by the NHS (➲ pages 199–207);
- social care provided by the local authority (➲ pages 193–98);
- personal care.

Personal care

This is the care that meets the personal needs of service users and involves assistance with:

- dressing, undressing, getting up and going to bed;
- personal hygiene – washing and bathing;
- toileting and continence management;
- nutrition – feeding and special diets;
- supporting mobility – by encouraging the use of mobility aids such as walking sticks, Zimmer frames and wheelchairs;
- assisting with medication;
- giving active support.

Active support

Active support for clients includes recognising diversity, promoting independence and choice, and treating clients with respect and dignity. It begins with listening carefully to the client and making an effort to understand what is being said. This is the first step in building up a good **client-carer relationship** to the benefit of both. The client will feel valued and have more confidence and trust in the carer, and the carer will get more job-satisfaction.

1. **a** Which people are in need of care?
   b Describe three different types of care.
   c What is involved in personal care?
   d What is involved in active support for clients?
   e What is the first step in building a good client-carer relationship?
   f What are the effects of a good carer-client relationship to the:
   i client,
   ii carer?

> ## Activity
> More and more people are being helped to remain in their own homes, even when they have very high health needs. Explain what personal care they may need.

Recognising diversity

Recognising diversity means regarding each service user as an individual with a family background, life history and personality that is unique and valuable. Clients often feel vulnerable (easily hurt) and treating them as individuals helps to improve their self-esteem and make them feel good about themselves. It takes time to build self-esteem and it is more likely to be achieved when a good relationship exists between client and carer. Clients will be more willing to cooperate and carers will find their job easier.

Promotion of independence and choice

This means encouraging clients and patients to be independent and to be involved in all decisions related to their care. Giving clients the freedom to make their own choices is an important aspect of caring. Failure to offer choices results in missed opportunities to promote clients' independence.

Treating individuals with respect and dignity

All service users, including children, should be treated with respect and dignity. This includes:

- listening to what they have to say, and replying in a kindly manner that does not offend them or damage their self-esteem;
- taking their requests seriously – if a request cannot be granted an explanation should be given;
- giving them the privacy and space they need;
- allowing them the right to practice their personal beliefs;
- respecting their right to confidentiality.

Protection

Clients and patients are often in a vulnerable position and many feel over-awed by the care professionals who are in charge. They therefore need protection from being:

- neglected, not listened to and ignored;
- harmed physically by maltreatment and abuse (➲ pages 47–8).

2. a What does recognising diversity mean?
   b What helps the self-esteem of vulnerable clients?
   c What does promotion of independence and choice mean?
   d What is the result of failing to offer choice to clients?
   e How are clients treated with respect and dignity?
   f What do clients need to be protected from?

Care assessment, plan and package

Care assessment is determining the needs of a client or patient, and is the first part of setting up a care plan. It can include:

- a medical assessment of the health of the client, which may include recommendations for the client's on-going care;
- an assessment of the client's skills for daily living;
- an assessment of the client's family on which to base long-term decisions for the client's care;
- an assessment of the home conditions.

Care plan

After the client or patient has been assessed, a care plan is put in writing that:

- describes the client's needs;
- decides the type of care needed;
- decides how the services will be provided;
- sets aims and goals for the client;
- monitors the way the plan is carried out;
- sets a date to review the plan.

Care package

When the amount of care needed has been assessed, a care package will be prepared. This can involve health and/or social care services and it shows how they will be paid for. At present, services provided by the NHS are free because the NHS pays for them. Services that are provided or arranged through the Social Services departments of local authorities are means-tested. A means test decides whether an applicant is able to pay for the services, and how much they have to pay.

Multi-disciplinary care

The care plan might involve multi-disciplinary care. This involves a range of health and social care professionals who work together to meet the needs of a client.

SAP (Single Assessment Process)

The SAP is used to reduce the number of assessments that are carried out on, for example, an older person, by different health and social care professionals. It forms the basis of a care plan.

3. a i What is care assessment?
   ii Describe four things that are assessed.
 b What does a care plan include?
 c What is involved in a care package?
 d What does multidisciplinary care involve?
 e Give an example of multidisciplinary care.

Activity

i Complete a SAP form and produce a care plan for the scenario on page 175.
ii Explain how meeting Dorothy's care needs can help to improve her self-concept (self-image and self-esteem).

A GP assesses the client's health.

A social worker assesses the client's care needs.

If necessary, a district nurse will provide nursing care.

Multi-disciplinary care

If necessary, a home carer will be provided.

An occupational therapist assesses the client's daily living skills.

Changing care needs at different stages of life

As individuals grow, develop and change, some of their needs stay the same and others alter. Needs that stay the same throughout life are food, water, shelter, safety, exercise, love and companionship, and health care.

Infancy (0-3 years)

Infants are completely dependent on their parents and carers to feed them and keep them warm, clean and safe. Love and affection from the adults who care for them builds strong bonds of attachment. These make them feel secure and valued, and helps them develop self-esteem. Infants also need space to play, toys for learning and practising skills, people to praise them as they learn and to teach them how to walk and talk. Child health clinics monitor their growth and development, and immunise them against childhood diseases.

Childhood (4-10 years)

Toys and space to play continue to be important to children's development. They are required to attend school where they are taught to read, write and use numbers. Families have the main responsibility for teaching them social skills and moral values.

Adolescence (11-18 years)

During the teenage years, adolescents become sexually mature and more independent and responsible for their own well-being. The **Health Promotion Services** offer advice to adolescents and adults about smoking, drugs, alcohol, contraception and sexually-transmitted diseases (STDs).

Adulthood (19-65 years)

Adulthood is a time of responsibility – for earning a living, providing a home, caring for children and, sometimes, for elderly parents. Adults may need help from:

- **Social Services** for housing, family support and counselling;
- **Citizens Advice** for help with legal and other problems;
- **Social Security** for income support;
- **Voluntary organisations** that provide specialist support when the family or one of its members is affected. For example, The Multiple Sclerosis Society, The Alzheimer's Society, Mencap and Gingerbread.

Activities

1. Explain the potential differences in care needs of individuals at different life stages from 0–65 years.
2. Four voluntary organisations are mentioned on this page. Briefly describe the purpose of each and where the nearest branch to you is situated. (➲ Media search page 245.)

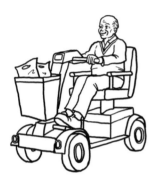

A **stair lift** makes it possible to get up and down stairs.

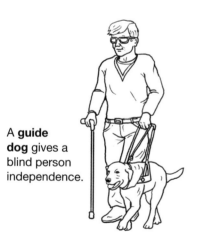

Scooters for people with walking difficulties makes it easier to get out and about.

A **guide dog** gives a blind person independence.

Activity

Go shopping with a person in a wheelchair. Report on any available facilities or difficulties that were encountered.

Older adults (65+)

As people get older they usually have fewer responsibilities and more leisure. But they are not as strong or as active as they used to be. Mobility (freedom and ease of movement) may become increasingly limited. Loneliness can also be a problem for those who are housebound or whose partner and friends have died.

Maintaining independence

Most people want to be independent for as long as possible. This can be achieved by:

- **health care**, for example mobility can be improved by pain relief, hip and knee joint replacements, and by help from a chiropodist (podiatrist) for care of the feet;
- **social care**, for example home carers to help with household tasks, meals-on-wheels, day centres and luncheon clubs to reduce loneliness, and volunteer drivers to help with transport;
- **disability aids**, two pieces of equipment are shown here but many more are available;
- **assistance dogs** – dogs trained to assist people with disabilities.

People with disabilities

People of any age with disabilities have the same basic needs for health and social care as everyone else in their age group. Their extra needs will depend on their particular disability.

Dogs for people with disabilities

Assistance dogs are trained to do tasks for people who find movement difficult. For example, picking up and fetching things, or help with dressing and undressing.

Hearing dogs These are assistance dogs for deaf people who are trained to make their owners aware of sounds such as the doorbell or phone.

4. **a** Give two physical changes that occur as people get older.
   b i What is mobility,
      ii how can health care improve mobility?
   c Name two pieces of equipment that assist mobility.
   d i Why may loneliness be a problem for older people,
      ii in what ways can social care help to reduce this?
   e Describe three types of assistance dogs.

Equipment for disabilities

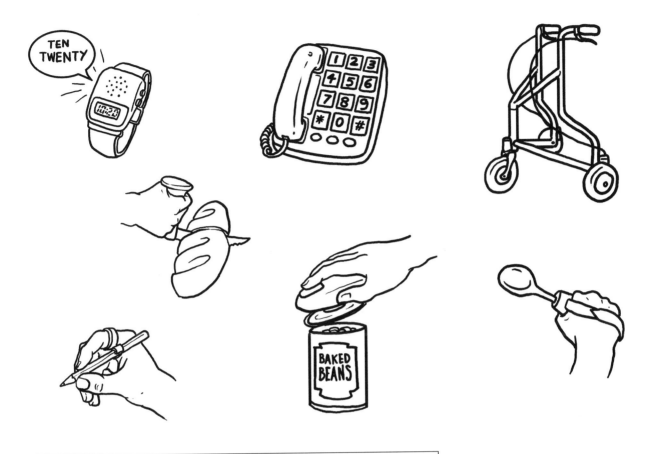

Scenario: Joe and Dorothy

Joe's wife Dorothy had always kept their house clean and tidy and she had always prided herself on her appearance. However, since Joe's accident at work, which left him paralysed down one side of the body and with the use of only one hand, Dorothy has not been able to find time to clean the house properly or go to the hairdressers regularly. She has become very depressed and her self-concept is very low. She no longer invites friends round for a meal and doesn't like to leave the house. The social worker, Karen, has assessed the needs of Joe and Dorothy and is writing a care plan for them. She has identified that Dorothy's self-image and self-esteem are very low and so her care plan includes actions designed to make time for Dorothy to go to the hairdresser, and to provide help for Dorothy to keep the house clean and tidy. Karen, Dorothy and Joe agree on a goal for Dorothy to invite close friends for a meal in three weeks' time.

5. In what ways could the equipment shown above be helpful to people with disabilities?

Activity

Research from at least two sources the equipment that would make Joe's life easier by improving his care needs and his self-concept. (See also the Activity on page 172 Regarding the assessment of Dorothy's needs.)

The final stages of life

Palliative care

Palliative care is a support system for those who are terminally ill and their families. It maintains quality of life by:

- providing relief from pain and other symptoms;
- helping patients live as actively as possible until death;
- offering a support system to help the family cope during the patient's illness;
- offering bereavement counselling to family and friends.

Hospice care

Hospices are places where staff and volunteers work in multi-disciplinary teams to offer freedom from pain, dignity, peace and calm at the end of life. They care for the person who is dying and their families in the hospice and at home. There is a range of services to meet all needs – physical, emotional, social – by offering nursing and medical care, counselling, complementary therapies, spiritual care, art, music, physiotherapy, beauty treatments and bereavement support.

Dying is a natural part of life. It is the process that a person goes through when all the systems in the body begin to slow down in the approach to death. A person who is dying needs to be kept free from pain and discomfort.

A person who is dying can be comforted by the presence of someone just to hold their hand and talk to them.

Activity

Explain the care needs of people in the final stages of life.

6. a What is palliative care?
   b What does palliative care do?
   c What happens in hospices?

Chapter 7
Creative and Therapeutic Activities

This chapter covers:

- An investigation of different creative and therapeutic activities appropriate to users in health and social care settings.

- Exploring the potential benefits of creative and therapeutic activities for service users.

- Examining the aspects of health and safety legislation, regulations and codes of practice that are relevant to the implementation of creative and therapeutic activities.

Creative and therapeutic activities

Creative activities aim to produce something original. **Therapeutic activities** aim to improve health and mobility. Many activities are both creative and therapeutic. When people are occupied, they feel more positive, feel less pain and depression, and can get pleasure from learning new skills and achieving something new.

In health and care settings these activities are used either as individual activities or in groups:

- to relax and relieve stress and boredom;
- for mental health problems;
- for those with learning difficulties;
- for children and young people with behaviour problems;
- for people with issues such as anger management;
- to improve physical health and mobility;
- to provide social contact for lonely people.

Health and care settings where creative and therapeutic activities take place

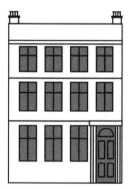

Community groups such as charities and voluntary groups.

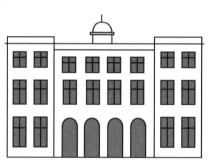

Hospitals – in children's wards and rehabilitation departments.

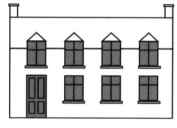

Day care centres for young children, elderly or disabled people.

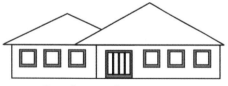

Care homes that provide residential care.

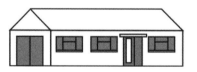

Domiciliary care – activities take place in service users' own homes.

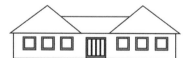

Pre-school care – play therapy in nurseries, play schools and family centres.

Activities

1. Visit at least two health or care settings when creative and/or therapeutic activities are taking place.
2. Invite a hospital play worker or an organiser of creative and therapeutic activities in a care setting to speak to your group.

Activities

Drama and role play

Both drama and role play are activities that involve interaction with other people, the need to listen attentively to others and to speak out clearly.

Drama

Taking part in a play requires team work and commitment, and can be both emotional and exciting.

Role play

Role play can be a short sketch in which the actors perform imaginary roles. Acting out a given situation such as a newspaper story means that each actor has to think like another person, imagine how they would react and what they would say. Role play is used in therapy:

- to help people understand the views of others by playing a role with a different point of view from their own;
- to help reduce anxiety caused by stressful situations such as preparation for an interview;
- to practice skills, for example parenting skills and **assertiveness skills** (the ability to express wishes and opinions in a firm and confident manner).

Photography

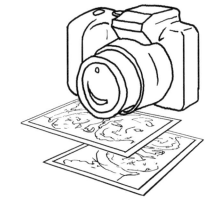

Photography is an activity for individuals or small groups. It can be done anywhere – indoors or outside. Taking photos involves:

- looking and thinking about the world outside yourself – at people, views from a window, scenery, birds, animals and flowers;
- deciding what pictures to take;
- seeing immediate results when a digital camera is used;
- using a computer to print photos from a digital camera;
- choosing photos to put in an album or for a wall display.

Activity

With another student, role play an organiser of health and therapeutic activities who is encouraging a service user to take up photography (or any other activity). Describe:
i the equipment needed and the decisions to be made,
ii the benefits for the service user.

Art and craft therapy

Arts and crafts are creative and absorbing. They require concentration and hand and finger control, provide opportunities to learn new skills or regain old skills, and are a basis for conversation. Successful completion of a project gives satisfaction and improves self-esteem.

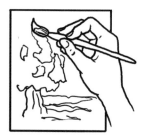

Painting and drawing
People who have been traumatised by real-life experiences may find it easier to unlock their feelings in pictures rather than by talking about them.

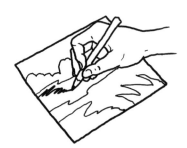

Colouring is a restful activity and results in a sense of accomplishment.

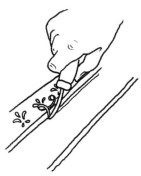

Leather craft is a very social activity and results can be achieved within an hour.

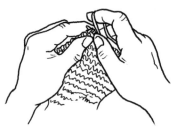

Knitting is an activity that one person can do on their own, when and where they please. Patterns can be simple or complicated and a useful article can be produced.

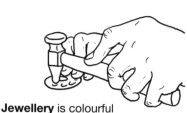

Jewellery is colourful and demands fine finger control.

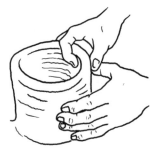

Modelling with clay or plaster of Paris uses the hands, provides the opportunity to be creative and encourages interaction with others.

Art therapy uses a wide variety of materials

Activities

1. Try out some arts and crafts activities. How did you feel about learning new skills and achieving results? Which service users might you recommend for each activity? Which service users might the activity not be suitable for?
2. Prepare an exhibition of arts and crafts made in health and care settings, or take photographs of them. Accompany each exhibit with a brief description of where the exhibit was made, why it was made and by whom (with the service user's permission). For example, a cane basket made at the rehabilitation clinic by a man who had a stroke and was trying to regain more use of his affected hand.

Music therapy

Music therapy is the use of music to encourage feelings of well-being, to relieve stress and to improve confidence of the listeners. It is used in many health and social care settings either with groups or on a one-to-one basis. The therapist and clients take an active part in the sessions by playing, singing or listening to music together.

Music has a powerful effect on the mind. Different kinds of music can result in different kinds of feelings including calmness, energy, release from unwanted thoughts, pleasure in reminiscence, irritation or anger. Music therapy is used:

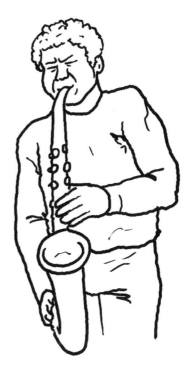

- for relaxation therapy in treatment for stress, insomnia, anxiety and depression;
- to improve breathing by playing wind instruments;
- to improve **manual dexterity** (hand control) by playing an instrument;
- to improve **motor skills** (muscle movements) by exercising or dancing to music;
- for physical rehabilitation in stroke victims;
- to encourage communication and shared pleasure by singing together or talking about different types of music and musicians;
- for reminiscence therapy – using tunes and songs from times past (➲ page 184).

Cooking therapy

Preparing food and cooking is a useful life skill and essential for people living on their own. It is a skill that occupational therapists assess to find out if people about to be discharged from hospital are capable of living at home on their own. It is an activity that can be done individually or with others in a cookery class.

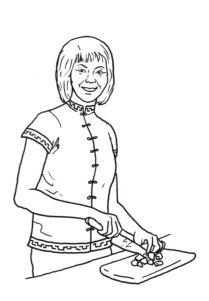

It can help to regain lost skills such as:

- making decisions – what to cook, which recipe, how to obtain the ingredients, how much to use;
- hand control when using knives and other implements;
- careful use of equipment such as kettles, saucepans and ovens to prevent burns;
- concentration to produce an end result;
- independence.

Activity

Find out more about music or cooking as therapy. Using text and images explain why each is a useful form of therapy.

Gardening therapy

Gardening is an activity that can help anyone with a disability. For example, it can:

- be used to rebuild strength after an accident or illness;
- relieve stress by providing a peaceful activity;
- help restore emotional well-being for a person going through a difficult time;
- give a sense of achievement in growing things;
- improve literacy and planning through reading a seed packet or looking at seed catalogues and gardening magazines;
- improve self-esteem.

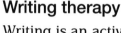

Activity

Read and summarise information from a document on gardening as therapy and a document on writing as therapy.
(➲ page 245 Media search.)

Gardening has made Jim more observant, improved the use of his hands, allowed him to be creative, to enjoy being out-of-doors, and taking exercise. He found greenery is very restful, scents from flowers are pleasing and producing fruit and vegetables is very satisfying.

Writing therapy

Writing is an activity that is usually done by people working on their own and can be used as therapy for people who have suffered traumatic, stressful or emotional events. Patients who write about their deepest thoughts and feelings can gain improvements in emotional health and happiness.

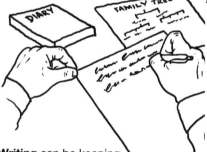

Writing can be keeping a diary or writing a story, autobiography, family history, a play or poetry.

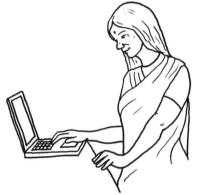

Using computers

Computers can be used for creative activities such as writing, obtaining information from the internet, playing games and printing photos. Using a computer encourages the hands and brain to become more agile.

Movement therapy

Movement therapy means taking exercise of one form or another. Exercise keeps muscles strong and joints mobile. People who find it very difficult to do routine exercises on their own often enjoy being part of a group.

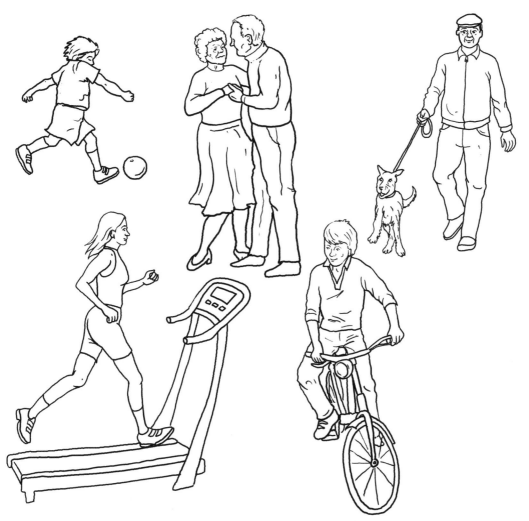

There are many ways of exercising

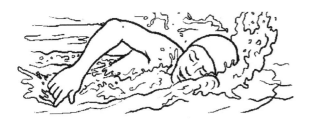

Activity

Use a questionnaire to find opinions on the therapeutic benefits of people taking different forms of exercise. Ask family and friends, patients and service users, health and social care professionals. Compare the results from each group you question. What are the similarities and differences? (➲ page 246 Questionnaires.)

Puzzles, games and quizzes

The brain, like all other parts of the body, deteriorates if it is not used. The activities shown here:

- help to keep the brain active;
- improve problem-solving;
- prevent boredom;
- are suitable for all ages and abilities;
- can be done individually, in pairs or in groups.

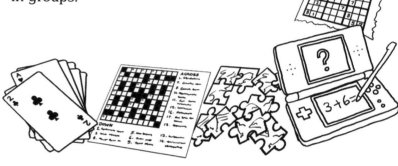

Reminiscence therapy

Reminiscence is thinking, talking or writing about the past. Besides being used to pass on information (usually to a new generation), reminiscence can also be used as therapy. For example, it can be used:

- to assist the recovery of memory in a patient with amnesia;
- to help the mental functioning of a patient with dementia;
- to relieve the stress of mourning, by remembering the pleasure of happy times (people remember happy times more readily than unhappy ones);
- as an enjoyable event in residential care.

In any health and social care setting individuals have the right to refuse to take part in reminiscence activities, and this right should be respected.

Memories are stimulated by

Old photographs, pictures and films.

Familiar tunes.

Familiar smells.

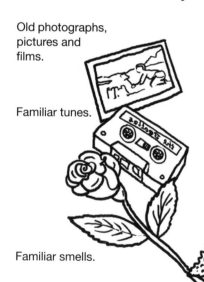

Touching objects and feeling textures.

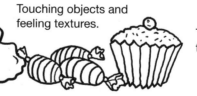

The sight and taste of foods.

Activity

With other students in your group, collect items for reminiscence therapy or for a session of games or a quiz. Organise an event when they can be used in a health or care setting. Produce a report of the occasion using either a computer or a tape recorder. Include your opinion on any benefits to those taking part.

Health and safety legislation

A number of health and safety laws apply to hospitals, care homes, clinics and other health and care settings. Their aim is to protect both the people who work there and the general public who use them. The laws are based on good management and the common sense that most employers and employees use anyway: that is, to look at what the risks are and take sensible measures to avoid them. For example:

- ensure that the workplace is as safe as possible;
- identify any hazards and potential risks;
- control exposure to chemicals and other hazardous substances to prevent ill-health;
- make proper use of equipment provided for safety;
- avoid the need for hazardous manual handling;
- report work-related accidents and diseases;
- ensure that food intended for human consumption is safe;
- take care of your own and others' safety at work;
- follow the hygiene regulations for food preparation and handling.

Laws relating to creative and therapeutic activities

The appropriate health and safety regulations must be followed when creative and therapeutic activities are carried out in health and care settings. For example:

- 'Health and Safety at Work Act 1974' (➲ page 54);
- 'Manual Handling Regulations 1992' (➲ page 56);
- 'Control of Substances Hazardous to Health Regulations (COSHH) 1994' (➲ page 55);
- 'Management of Health and Safety at Work Regulations 1999' and 'Risk assessment' (➲ page 54);
- 'Reporting Injuries, Diseases and Dangerous Occurrences Regulations (RIDDOR) 1995' (➲ page 56);
- 'Food Safety Act 1990' (➲ page 239);
- 'Food Safety (General Food Hygiene) Regulations 1992' (➲ page 239).

Wash hands before eating.

Use a face mask for activities that produce dust.

Wipe up spilt liquid.

Open windows when fumes are produced.

Sink for washing paintbrushes.

Lead in paint can be poisonous.

Report accidents in the 'accidents book'.

Examples of health and safety measures

Activity

For each of the activities named in your plans for individual patients or service users (➲ page 187):

a identify the sensible measures you need to take;
b carry out a risk assessment (➲ page 54);
c identify the relevant legislation;
d make notes of any health and safety instructions to be given to those carrying out the activities.

Benefits of creative and therapeutic activities

Creative and therapeutic activities can help patients and clients to ignore pain or disabilities, problems or worries. Depending on individual needs, these activities are also used to:

- maintain current skills, improve them, develop new skills or regain lost skills;
- reduce boredom;
- help with emotional problems and depression;
- improve mobility and fitness;
- improve **dexterity** – ability in using the hands and fingers;
- develop the imagination and improve problem solving;
- develop communication skills and improve speech;
- improve self-esteem – this comes with achievements such as painting a picture, baking a cake or knitting a scarf – if the patient/client is pleased with the result and it is admired by others, so much the better;
- improve cooperation and develop friendships;
- promote independence by encouraging **coping strategies** – learning how to live with difficult lifestyle changes.

The potential benefits and therapeutic value of an activity depend on several factors:

- the age of the person;
- gender;
- health;
- mobility;
- social and cultural background;
- the service user's preferences.

Activities

1. From the list of benefits name:
   - one physical benefit;
   - two intellectual benefits;
   - two language benefits;
   - two emotional benefits;
   - two social benefits;
   - other benefits not included in the answers above.
2. Explaining the benefits, suggest two activities suitable for people with:
   - weakness in one side of the body;
   - loss of an arm;
   - memory loss;
   - boredom;
   - loss of the ability to speak;
   - separation from loved ones;
   - grief;
   - depression;
   - new living arrangements;
   - loneliness.
3. Compare your answers with those of other students.

Planning creative/therapeutic activities for individual patients/service users in a health and care setting

1. Initial draft

- Choose a patient or service user, and explain why you chose that person.
- Select an activity and explain why it was chosen.
- Research the activity, identify the materials needed and the quantity of the materials.
- Select the date, time and place for you to observe, and take part in, the activity with your chosen individual.
- Identify the relevant legislation, regulations and codes of practice that apply to the safety of everyone involved, patients/service users, yourself and others.
- Identify the potential benefits of the activity to the patient/service user.
- Show the initial draft to the assessor.

2. Produce a final plan

- Write a final plan including a step-by-step guide for setting up the activity – time, place, access, heating, lighting, materials and equipment needed for the activity.

3. Carry out the activity

- Ideally, ask an appropriate staff member in the health or social care setting to complete a witness statement as additional evidence.

4. Evaluate the activity

- Explain how the creative/therapeutic activity could benefit the patient/service user.
- Recommend ways of improving the activity, taking into account individual needs of the patient/service user.
- Describe how the health and safety issues of the activity were addressed.
- Explain why it was necessary to implement the specific health and safety measures, linking the measures to the laws, regulations and codes of practice.

5. Plan a second activity

- Carry out steps 1-4 above for a different patient or service user with a different activity.

6. Discuss your plans with other students.

Occupational Therapy (OT)

Registered occupational therapists (often called OTs) help people of all ages to overcome the effects of disability caused by physical or mental illness, ageing or accident. OTs enable these disabled patients to lead full and satisfying lives, living as independently as possible, by assessing the needs of each patient, and then designing a programme of treatment for them.

Occupational therapists work in hospitals, health centres, social services departments, residential homes and day centres. They also visit clients in their own homes, and assist others with rehabilitation.

Rehabilitation

Rehabilitation helps people who have been ill or are disabled to return to normal life. Occupational therapists encourage individuals to take action for themselves by advising on:

- **personal care** – how to wash and dress, brush the teeth, use the toilet and go shopping;
- **work** – how to continue with housework or unpaid jobs;
- **employment** – talking with employers to see if the employee's usual work can be adapted to their new disabilities so that they can return to work;
- **leisure activities** – how to take part in hobbies, sport or other social activities;
- **social life** – how to find satisfactory ways of meeting people if they are unable to work;
- **home adaptations** – making recommendations on simple changes to the home to make life easier, such as grip assists in the kitchen for taps, hand utensils and kettle-pouring;
- **specialist equipment** – advising on wheelchairs and stair lifts to improve independence;
- **psychological attitudes** to help regain morale following illness or injury – this may include working with the family and carers;
- **education** – giving advice about continuing with education while coping with illness or disability.

Activities

1. Invite an Occupational Therapist to speak to your group, or watch a video (from the internet) of their work.
2. Use the internet to find out how to become a registered occupational therapist:
   i the qualifications needed to start training,
   ii the qualifications received when training is complete.
3. **Disabled Living Foundation (DLF)** is a national charity helping older and disabled people to find equipment that helps them to lead independent lives. Investigate their website (**www.dlf.org.uk**) to find out what the organisation offers.

Chapter 8

Health and Social Care Services

This chapter covers:

- The organisation of health and social care provision.

- The benefits of working in partnership for health and social care provision.

- Working in the health and social care sectors.

Health and social work provision

A hundred years ago, people who were poor or sick were fortunate if they received charity from churches, voluntary organisations or wealthy individuals. Hospitals were built and maintained by donations and conditions in them varied widely. A consultation with a doctor usually required payment. There were no old-age pensions, child allowances, unemployment benefits or help for large families. People in need were usually dependent on any care that family, friends or neighbours could give. Today, health and social care is provided in various ways by the statutory, private and voluntary services and by informal care from family, friends and neighbours.

Statutory services

These are services provided by the state and include the National Health Service (NHS) and Social Services. They are set up by government statutes (laws) and most of their services are free. The money to run them comes from the taxes we all pay in one form or another.

Private services

These services charge fees. Examples are private hospitals, nursing homes, private care homes, private doctors and dentists, childminders and most complementary therapy.

Voluntary services

These are **Not-for-Profit Organisations** such as **charities** and they are staffed partly, or in some cases completely, by volunteers. Money to run them is raised from charity shops, flag days and a great variety of other fund-raising events. The money is then used for the benefits that the charity provides. Voluntary organisations vary in size from the very large such as the NSPCC, Cancer Research UK and Age Concern, to smaller groups such as the Zipper Club (for heart surgery patients), Cruse (for the bereaved), Macmillan Cancer Support and Marie Curie Cancer Care to the many small local charity groups.

1. **a** Name two services provided by the state.
   b Which of the three types of services are:
   i   not-for-profit,
   ii provided by the state,
   iii privately owned,
   iv mostly free,
   v   charge fees,
   vi dependant on volunteer helpers?

Activities

1. Find out about the voluntary organisations in your area that provide different aspects of health and social care. Some you may already know, others may be advertised in newspapers, doctors' surgeries or Yellow Pages. Mark their positions on your street map (➲ page 4).
2. Describe the health care services, social care services and voluntary services that are provided where you live, and say what each does. (This could be based on your street map ➲ page 4.)

Statutory, private and voluntary services

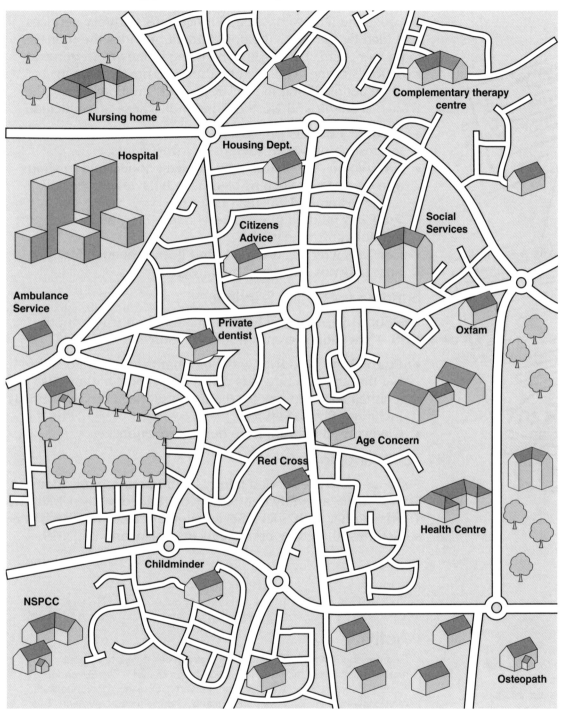

2. Copy the table below then place the services named on the plan into the appropriate column (5 in each group).

Statutory services	Private services	Voluntary services
1		
2		
3		
4		
5		

How the statutory services are funded

Because the NHS and Social Services are statutory services provided by the state, the government provides the money to pay for them. This is done by using money from **general taxation** – money collected by the government from taxes paid by people living in the UK (United Kingdom – England, Wales, Scotland and Northern Ireland). These taxes include:

- **Income Tax** paid on wages and salaries, and on the interest gained from savings or investments;
- **VAT** (Value-Added Tax) paid on most goods sold in shops and on services such as electricity bills, telephone calls, hairdressing and car repairs;
- **Fuel Tax** paid on petrol, diesel and oil for motor transport and for central heating;
- **Car Tax**, which is the road fund licence needed for cars, buses, lorries, vans and motor cycles.

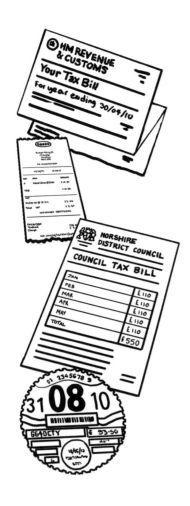

Funding for Social Services

The Social Services are funded in a different way from the NHS. Their money comes from two sources:

- **Council tax** paid by owners or tenants for each house or flat that they occupy. It is collected by local authorities (councils) to help pay for the many services run by councils including Social Services.
- **Government grants** from general taxation.

Joint funding

Some services are funded jointly by different organisations. For example, a Family Centre may be funded by the Children's Trust together with Social Services, and Cancer Research is sometimes funded by both a cancer charity and the NHS.

3. **a** Name four types of general taxation.
   b How is the NHS funded?
   c How are the Social Services funded?
   d **i** What is joint funding?
   ii Give an example.
   e Of the four taxes mentioned above, which have you paid recently, or have been paid by someone else on your behalf?

Activity

Find out about William Beveridge so that you can give a talk about him for at least four minutes. The report he produced – *The Beveridge Report* – identified 'five evils' of Want (poverty), Disease, Ignorance (lack of education), Squalor (poor housing) and Idleness (unemployment). This report led to the creation of the welfare state in Britain.

Social Care

Social care is the support for people who need help to meet their personal and social needs, but not their medical needs. It covers a wide range of services provided by:

- **Social Services** – the Local Authority (council) services;
- **private services**;
- **voluntary organisations**.

Each of these service providers deliver care through a number of different organisations, some of which are named below.

Citizens Advice

Fostering

Children's homes

Day centres

Young offenders

Samaritans

Salvation Army

Residential homes

Adoption

Youth work

Night shelters

Sheltered housing

Child protection

Home carers

Homeless families

Meals on wheels

British Legion

Princes Trust for young people

Organisations that provide social care

Activities

Use the internet to find answers to these questions.
1. The **Citizens Advice Bureau** helps people with their problems. Find out what types of problems.
2. Find out what the **Samaritans** provide and how to get in touch with them.
3. The **Salvation Army** is one of the largest providers of social services in the UK. Give at least ten examples of the wide range of services supported by this charity.
4. The **British Legion** cares for ex-service people. When does the annual Poppy Appeal take place, why does it take place and what are the funds used for?

1. **a** What is social care?
   b Name the three services that provide social care.
   c Eighteen organisations that provide social care are named on this page. Sort them into groups that provide care for:
   i babies and children (four groups),
   ii young people (three groups),
   iii older people (four groups),
   iv housing (three groups),
   v voluntary organisations (four groups).

Social Services

Social Services provide welfare services for people at times when they need care and support. Their clients include:

- children and families;
- older people;
- people with disabilities;
- people with learning difficulties;
- people with sensory impairments (blindness or deafness);
- people with mental health problems;
- people with drug or alcohol problems.

Partnership working

When a client's needs are complex, as they often are, Social Services work in partnership with other organisations to decide on the best course of action for that individual client. (➲ page 218–20.)

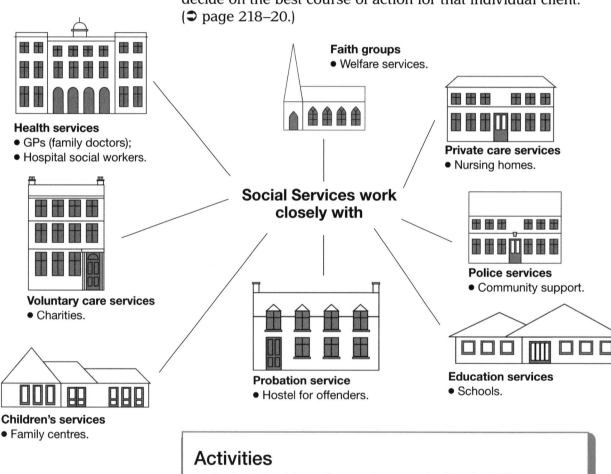

Health services
- GPs (family doctors);
- Hospital social workers.

Voluntary care services
- Charities.

Children's services
- Family centres.

Faith groups
- Welfare services.

Social Services work closely with

Probation service
- Hostel for offenders.

Private care services
- Nursing homes.

Police services
- Community support.

Education services
- Schools.

2. a i What is the purpose of Social Services,
ii who do their clients include?
b Which organisations do Social Services work closely with?

Activities

1. Find out about the welfare services organised by Social Services in your area (➲ Media search page 245).
2. Complete a chart of the organisations that Social Services work closely with and give examples of how they work together.

Social Services work closely with:	
Organisation	**Example**

Working in social care

Social workers

Social workers are qualified professionals who help people with personal, emotional or financial problems. They work alongside other professionals such as doctors to ensure that clients receive the support they need. A social worker's job involves:

- listening to clients;
- assessing clients' needs;
- providing information and advice;
- organising support services for clients;
- putting clients in touch with other agencies.

Anyone wishing to become a social worker cannot start training until they are 21 years old. Before then, students are encouraged to take jobs in social care organisations to gain experience of the work. When qualified with a Degree in Social Work they may wish to specialise in a particular area such as children and child protection, mental health, the elderly, youth and community services, or as a hospital social worker.

Activity

Interview a social care worker to find out what they do during a typical day at work. Write a report or record your interview on audio or video recorder.

Social care workers

Social care workers offer personal care in the tasks of everyday living. They may not need a qualification when they take on the job, and will usually work under the direction of a qualified social care worker or nurse. They will then be expected to work towards a qualification and may receive training by their employers to this end.

Most jobs for social care workers occur in three main areas:

- **domiciliary care** – people being looked after in their own homes by **home carers** (domiciliary care assistants);
- **residential homes**;
- **day care**.

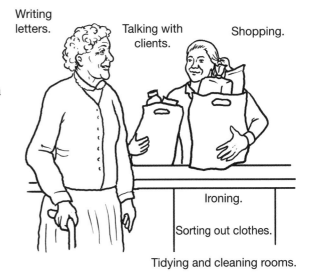

Writing letters. Talking with clients. Shopping. Ironing. Sorting out clothes. Tidying and cleaning rooms.

A home carer in action

3. **a** What are the differences between the job of a social worker and a social care worker?
   b **i** What does a social worker's job involve?
   ii at what age can training start,
   iii how can experience be gained before then?
   c What qualification does a social worker need?
   d What are the specialist areas of social work?
   e Is a qualification necessary for social care workers?
   f Name the main areas for jobs in social care work.
   g In what ways do home carers help their clients?

Residential homes

Residential homes provide permanent homes for people who cannot continue living in their own homes, even with the support from home carers. They cater for different client groups. There are children's homes, homes for the elderly and homes for those with physical or learning disabilities. Usually, no professional medical staff are employed at the home, but a GP (doctor) is on call if required. Care of the residents is undertaken by care assistants.

Care assistants help the residents:

- with washing, bathing, dressing and toileting;
- by preparing drinks and light snacks for them;
- by helping them with feeding and walking if necessary;
- by talking to them and by keeping an eye on their general condition.

Day centres

Day centres are care settings that people attend during the day, perhaps for five days a week, or just for one or two days. They provide opportunities to meet other people, to have a cooked lunch, to get involved with a variety of social activities, and for a change of scene for those who have difficulty in getting out. Services such as hairdressing and chiropody may be available, and there is an opportunity to have a supervised bath (for safety). Transport to and from the centre is usually arranged for those with mobility difficulties.

Care assistants in a day centre help clients by:

- welcoming them to the centre;
- helping them to order lunch;
- talking to them about their lives and interests;
- providing interesting activities for them to take part in.

Respite care

Respite care provides a short break for clients and their carers. Clients have a change of scene and contact with different people. Carers have a short break from their caring role. Respite can take the form of a few hours a day at a day centre, or a few days or a weekend or a couple of weeks. Many residential homes offer respite care.

4. a Explain the difference between a residential home, a day centre and respite care.
   b Name different types of residential care.
   c What is the purpose of day centres?
   d What do the care assistants in a day centre do?
   e Give a benefit of respite care for:
      i the clients,
      ii their carers.

Vacancies

Required

Manager for a residential home

As the manager you would be responsible for the day-to-day running of the home. Your duties would include:

- providing advice and support for the residents and their families;
- recruiting, training and supervising the care assistants and domestic staff;
- ensuring that the quality of the service and the care meets the National Standards;
- working within a budget and taking responsibility for the accounts.

Wanted

Mobile meals drivers

The council provides a hot meal service from Monday to Friday, and pre-packed frozen meals at the weekends and Bank Holidays. Meals are prepared in a central kitchen, and the hot meals packed in heat-retaining boxes. They are collected by volunteer drivers and delivered to clients between 11.15 am and 1 pm. This service:

- provides a value-for-money hot nutritional midday meal for elderly residents in the borough who are unable to provide one for themselves;
- improves the quality of life for the customers;
- ensures daily contact with the clients and a check on their well-being.

'Meals On Wheels' drivers are of all ages and from all walks of life, and drive their own cars. A full, clean driving licence is required, training is given and a mileage allowance is provided. Besides doing a very worthwhile job, drivers have the opportunity to meet new people.

Vacancy

Assistant youth worker

As a youth worker, your job would be to work with young people aged 13 to 19 years. You would provide enjoyable, educational and challenging activities to help them improve their confidence, develop new skills and cope with issues that affect their lives. The job could involve:

- organising sports, arts, drama, and other activities;
- mentoring and counselling;
- working with specific groups such as young carers or those at risk of offending;
- networking with other professionals including social workers, teachers, probation officers and the police.

Train to be a counsellor

A counsellor talks to people with personal problems, giving them time and attention with the assurance that all topics covered will remain confidential. The main purpose is not to give advice but to help them explore their thoughts, feelings and behaviour. Most counsellors work in a particular field such as marriage guidance, addiction, sexual abuse, domestic violence or bereavement. Counselling is usually done on a one-to-one basis and involves:

- building a relationship of trust and respect with the client;
- encouraging the client to talk about the feelings that have made them seek counselling;
- listening carefully and asking questions that enable you to understand the client's situation;
- helping the client to see things more clearly or from different points of view;
- referring the client to other sources of help, if appropriate;
- keeping confidential records.

New post

Care arranger

We are looking to recruit a full-time care arranger to join the team based at the council offices. Care arrangers act as a bridge between the purchasing teams and the domiciliary care providers. They are responsible for finding, agreeing and coordinating care for clients. The successful applicant will need computer skills, have a good telephone manner and be able to work to timescales.

The successful applicant will also need to have a good knowledge of the domiciliary care as well as to be able to establish and maintain good working relationships with a variety of professional people and organisations.

Community Development Worker

Community development workers work with individuals, families or the whole community to bring about social change and improve quality of life.

Job description and entry requirements
www.prospects.ac.uk

Family support worker

Family support workers provide emotional and practical help and advice to families who are experiencing short-term or long-term difficulties. They aim to help children (who may otherwise be taken into care) to stay with their families.

For further information contact:
careersadvice.direct.gov.uk

Activity

Investigate a job in social care that you might like to do.
i   Describe the requirements of the job,
ii Describe the skills needed for the job,
iii Explain why the requirements for the job are necessary.
   (➲ Writing a report page 242.)

5. Which of the seven jobs advertised on pages 197-8 do you find most attractive and least attractive. Give your reasons.

Health Care Services

Health care services exist to advise people on how to keep healthy and to treat people who are ill. When feeling unwell, there is the choice of:

- natural recovery – the body has great capacity for healing itself from many simple physical ailments if given time, and emotional problems can be helped by rest, relaxation, a change of occupation or a holiday;
- advice from relatives or friends;
- advice or medication by using one or more of the options below.

Self care →	A well-stocked, lockable medicine cabinet can help with many of the more common illnesses.
Pharmacist →	The local pharmacist is qualified to give advice on the treatment of many ailments.
NHS Direct →	Free, confidential health advice can be obtained, 24 hours a day, by telephoning the helpline, which in England is 0845 4647.
NHS Direct Online →	Health advice and information about hundreds of illnesses and self-help groups is available on the internet: **nhsdirect.nhs.uk**
NHS Walk-in Centre →	An experienced nurse and/or a doctor treats minor injuries and illnesses, seven days a week, early until late.
GP's Surgery →	Patients who are registered with a GP can make an appointment to see a doctor or practice nurse.
A & E or Ambulance Service →	Call 999/112 or visit the nearest Accident and Emergency Department for emergency or urgent care.

Activities

1. Check the medicine cabinet at home or elsewhere. List its contents, find out what each medicine is for, when it expires and suggest other items that would be useful.
2. Compare the NHS Direct helplines in England with those in Wales, Scotland and Northern Ireland – the telephone number to call, when to contact, the service provided, etc.

1. **a** What personal actions can help speed recovery?
   b When needing medical advice or treatment, where could you go for:
   i to make an appointment;
   ii advice on the telephone;
   iii medicines for common ailments;
   iv treatment for minor injuries;
   v treatment for emergencies;
   vi advice on the internet.

Structure of the NHS

The function of the NHS is to improve the health and well-being of the population. When it was set up in 1948, the same conditions applied to all the countries in the UK – England, Wales, Scotland and Northern Ireland. Following the reforms of 1997, differences have developed between the countries. In this section we will discuss the organisation of the NHS in England.

Activity

Compare the NHS England with NHS Scotland, NHS Wales or NHS Northern Ireland. Draw a diagram similar to the one on this page to show the structure of the NHS in that country. (◕ Media search page 245.)

NHS in England

Department of Health

This is the government department that provides the money for the NHS and gives overall directions on how it should be spent.

Strategic Health Authorities (SHAs)

There are ten Strategic Health Authorities each responsible for an area of England. Their function is to improve the health services in that area and to make sure that they are performing well. The health services are divided into primary care and secondary care.

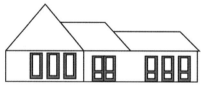

Health Centre

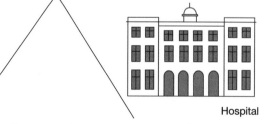

Hospital

Primary care services

Primary care is the term used for the health services that are provided in the community. It is called 'primary care' because it is usually the first point of contact that patients have with the NHS. Primary care is mainly concerned with general health needs and covers services provided by GPs and Health Centres.

Secondary care services

Secondary care is the term used for health care given in hospitals and the more specialised services such as ambulances and health care for the mentally ill. Arrangements for patients to receive secondary care are usually made by the GPs and other primary care services.

2. **a** When was the NHS set up?
   b When did each country in the UK become responsible for its own NHS?
   c Who controls NHS England?
   d How many SHAs are there?
   e Name the two divisions of the health service.
   f Explain the difference between primary care and secondary care.

NHS Trusts

The NHS contains many organisations called 'Trusts'. The Trusts run the different parts of the NHS at local level, providing services for patients in the community and in hospitals. They are responsible for providing most of the health and community care for millions of people in the UK, and they use up about three-quarters of the NHS budget. Trusts are a part of both primary care and secondary care.

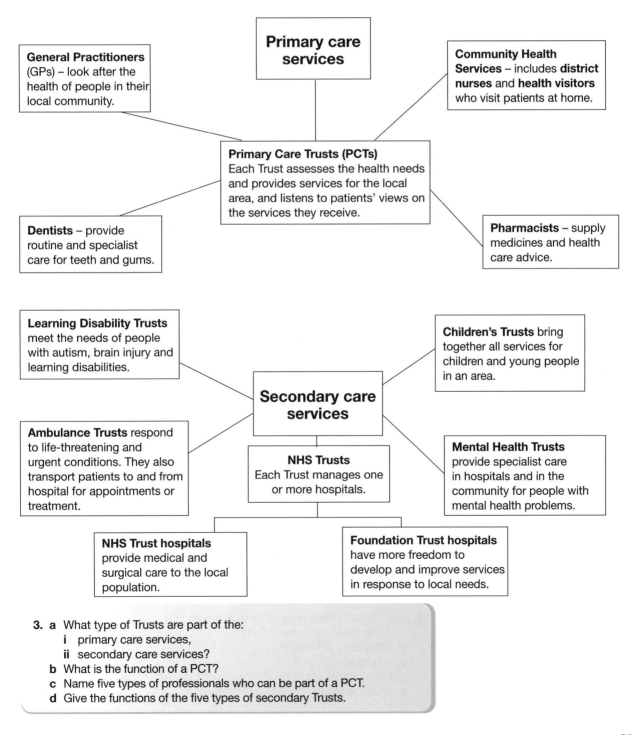

General Practitioners (GPs) – look after the health of people in their local community.

Primary care services

Community Health Services – includes **district nurses** and **health visitors** who visit patients at home.

Primary Care Trusts (PCTs)
Each Trust assesses the health needs and provides services for the local area, and listens to patients' views on the services they receive.

Dentists – provide routine and specialist care for teeth and gums.

Pharmacists – supply medicines and health care advice.

Learning Disability Trusts meet the needs of people with autism, brain injury and learning disabilities.

Children's Trusts bring together all services for children and young people in an area.

Secondary care services

Ambulance Trusts respond to life-threatening and urgent conditions. They also transport patients to and from hospital for appointments or treatment.

NHS Trusts
Each Trust manages one or more hospitals.

Mental Health Trusts provide specialist care in hospitals and in the community for people with mental health problems.

NHS Trust hospitals provide medical and surgical care to the local population.

Foundation Trust hospitals have more freedom to develop and improve services in response to local needs.

3. **a** What type of Trusts are part of the:
   i primary care services,
   ii secondary care services?
   b What is the function of a PCT?
   c Name five types of professionals who can be part of a PCT.
   d Give the functions of the five types of secondary Trusts.

Primary care

Most primary care is centred on a medical practice staffed with a team of people that typically includes:

- **GPs** (**general practitioners**), often called family doctors – GPs deal with a variety of illnesses and complaints;
- **practice nurses** – qualified nurses who work with the doctors in the medical practice as part of a team;
- **practice managers**;
- **medical receptionists**;
- **community health nurses**;
- **dentists**.

The team may also include pharmacists, secretarial assistants and health care assistants.

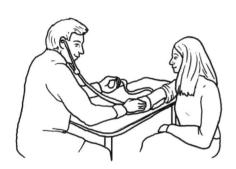

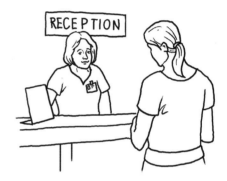

GP taking a patient's blood pressure. GPs listen to a patient's problems, check the medical condition and **diagnose** (identify an illness). Treatment may then be prescribed, further investigations carried out, or the patient referred to a hospital for specialist advice.

A medical receptionist makes appointments, answers the telephone and monitors the flow of people into the **consulting room** (where the doctor sees patients) and the **treatment room** (where the doctor or nurse gives treatments).

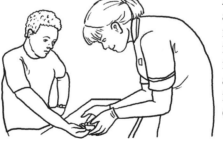

A practice nurse dressing a patient's hand. Practice nurses have many skills including wound care, giving immunisations, sexual health advice and clinics for long-term illnesses such as asthma and diabetes.

Activity

Describe a visit to see your GP at the health centre or doctor's practice.

i   How did you make an appointment?
ii Which member of staff did you meet first?
iii Describe the waiting room.
iv Find out who are employed in the health centre/practice and the jobs that they do.

4. a i What is most primary care centred on?
     ii who may the team include?
   b What does GP mean?
   c Who is a practice nurse?
   d Compare the job of a GP with that of a practice nurse.
   e Describe the job of a medical receptionist.

Community health care

Community health care is carried out by nurses. They see patients in health centres, family centres and clinics, or they visit patients in their own homes.

A **health visitor** is a qualified nurse or midwife who has further qualifications in the promotion of health and the prevention of illness. Much of their time is spent visiting people in their own homes. They advise mothers of young babies on aspects of childcare, and people who suffer from chronic illness or disability on ways of coping with the difficulties they face.

A **district nurse** cares for patients in their own homes or in residential homes. Patients may include those who are housebound, the elderly or disabled, or those recently discharged from hospital.

Community psychiatric nurses are trained nurses specialising in mental disorders. They visit patients at home and meet them at day centres and drop-in clinics.

Community midwives attend the births of babies born at home. Midwives are nurses who are specially trained to look after mothers and their babies before, during and after the birth. Their work includes antenatal and postnatal clinics.

The **practice manager** is responsible for staff rotas, buying supplies, paying the bills, producing accounts and many other duties.

Activities

1. Find out how to become a nurse – the qualifications needed to become a student nurse, where the training takes place, the time it requires, and the options open to qualified nurses.
2. Investigate a job in nursing that you might like to do.
   i   Describe the requirements of the job.
   ii Describe the skills needed for the job role.
   iii Explain why the requirements for the job are necessary.
   (➲ Writing a report page 242.)

5. a Which of the nurses working in the primary care services:
   i   works mainly with young families;
   ii gives domiciliary care;
   iii specialises in mental disorders;
   iv gives antenatal care.
   b What does the practice manager do?

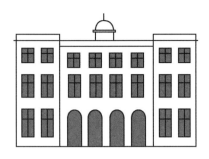

Secondary health care

Hospitals

Secondary care takes place mainly in hospitals. A large number of people are employed to do the many different jobs that require all types of skills and qualifications. A hospital is divided into departments, each specialising in treating a particular area of ill-health.

Different departments in a hospital

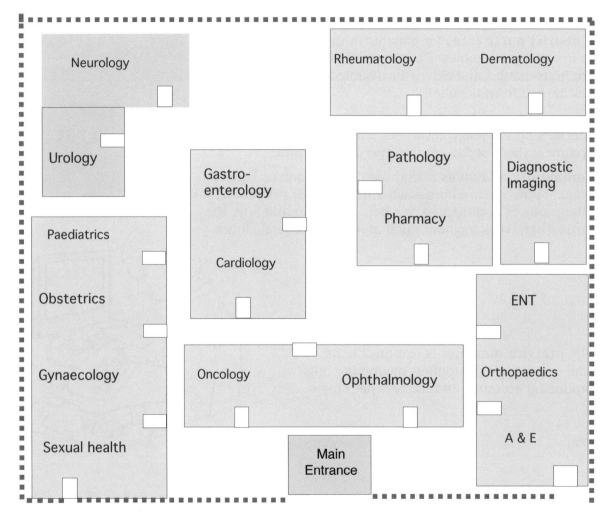

Activity

Visit a hospital:

i   describe the main reception area and what happens there,

ii make a list of the different jobs that people have in the hospital's reception area,

iii make a note of how you felt about the hospital – was it welcoming, frightening, comforting, reassuring?

6. From your own knowledge, or using a dictionary, which of the 18 hospital departments above specialises in:

blood	gonorrhoea	accidents/emergencies
heart	medicines	kidneys and bladder
skin	X-rays and scans	pregnancy and birth
cancer	muscles and joints	stomach and intestines
bones	nervous system	ear, nose and throat
children	female organs	eyes and sight

Hospital staff

Doctors

Medical students undergo several years of training and pass many examinations before they obtain a medical qualification and can become a doctor. They then decide whether to specialise as a GP and work in the community, become a hospital doctor or enter public health or full-time administration.

Hospital doctors spend a number of years specialising in one particular branch of medicine in order to become a **consultant** (specialist doctor), such as a physician, surgeon, paediatrician, gynaecologist, radiologist and pathologist.

Nurses

Nurses are trained to care for people who are sick and to carry out some medical and surgical procedures. When student nurses become qualified as Registered Nurses, they can choose to work in every sort of health care setting, for example:

- hospitals, perhaps specialising in one of the many departments such as accident and emergency, diabetes, children's nursing, mental health nursing, intensive care or as an operating theatre nurse;
- nursing homes;
- health centres;
- patients' homes;
- a military nursing service.

Health care assistants

Health care assistants (sometimes called nursing auxiliaries or auxiliary nurses) work alongside nurses and midwives. They are an important part of the nursing team in hospitals and other health care settings such as nursing homes and care homes. They carry out general duties for patients such as:

- recording temperature, pulse rate, breathing rate and blood pressure;
- helping patients to wash, bathe or shower;
- assist patients with toileting;
- serving food and, if necessary, helping patients to eat;
- making and changing beds;
- keeping the ward tidy;
- talking with patients to help them feel less lonely or anxious.

Activity

Find out how to become a health care assistant.

7. **a** Name the six types of specialist doctor that are mentioned on this page.
   b What are nurses trained to do but not health care assistants?
   c Name three types of care settings that employ health care assistants.
   d What are the general duties of a health care assistant?

Pharmacists (sometimes called chemists) are experts in medicines and their use. They are qualified and registered health professionals who are trained to:

- dispense medicines;
- give advice on their proper use;
- give advice on minor ailments;
- advise on healthy living, for example, how to give up smoking.

Radiographers take images (pictures) of the inside of the body to help in the diagnosis of disease by using:

- radiation for X-rays, CT scans and radio isotopes;
- magnetism for MRI scans (magnetic resonance imaging);
- ultra-sound waves for ultrasound scans.

Speech and language therapists work with people who have problems with communication including speech defects, and with chewing or swallowing.

Chiropodists (Podiatrists) treat disorders of the feet and ankles. They work to improve mobility and relieve pain. They help patients to walk more easily and maintain their independence.

Health professionals

Health professionals are people who work closely with doctors in the treatment of disease. They do not have a medical degree, but have qualifications in their own speciality. In addition to those described on this page, medical professionals include:

- physiotherapists (⊃ pages 98–9);
- occupational therapists (⊃ page 188);
- dietitians (⊃ page 235);
- psychologists (⊃ page 127).

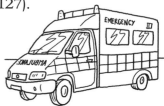

Ambulance crews that respond to 999/112 calls are trained in emergency care and decide whether to treat patients at the scene or transport them to hospital.

- **Paramedics** are crew members highly-trained in emergency medical procedures. They use high-tech equipment, such as that needed for heart attacks, to give intravenous drips and administer medicines and oxygen. Their actions can greatly increase a patient's chances of recovery.
- **Ambulance care assistants** transport patients to and from hospitals.

Medical technicians are involved in the operation and maintenance of high-tech equipment such as body scanners.

Activity

Find out how to become a doctor or other medical professional.
i   Describe the requirements of the job,
ii describe the skills needed for the job,
iii explain why the requirements for the job are necessary.
(⊃ Writing a report page 242.)

8. **a** Who are medical professionals?
   b Which medical professionals:
   i help people with a stutter, **ii** dispense medicines,
   iii treat disorders of the feet, **iv** advise on diet,
   v maintain high-tech equipment, **vi** take X-rays,
   vii help the body to recover after injury?
   c Explain the difference between an ambulance care assistant and a paramedic.
   d What are the following used for in the diagnosis of disease?
   i radiation, **ii** magnetism, **iii** ultra sound waves.
   e Give another name for a podiatrist.

Hospital support services

Many large hospitals that serve a wide area are likely to have a number of facilities for the well-being of patients and their visitors. These include hospital chaplains, non-medical staff and hospital volunteers.

Hospital chaplains

Hospitals can be stressful places and hospital chaplains provide support for patients, families and staff. They listen to personal problems and give confidential advice and spiritual support. Chaplains of different religious faiths visit the wards and talk with the patients. If the hospital has a chapel, religious services will be held for patients, visitors and staff who wish to attend. Many hospitals offer a bereavement service where information and support is offered to the relatives and friends of someone who has died.

Non-medical staff

People employed in a hospital but do not have direct care for patients include:

managers,	office staff,
housekeepers,	catering staff,
medical secretaries,	cleaning staff,
medical social workers,	porters,
electricians,	plumbers.

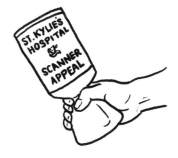

Hospital volunteers

Although NHS hospitals are paid for out of taxes, there is never enough money to pay for everything a hospital needs, and voluntary help is much appreciated. These unpaid helpers assist in many ways by:

- carrying out routine tasks for the staff on the wards;
- running errands for patients, writing letters or shopping;
- helping in reception by directing patients or visitors to the right clinic or ward, or assisting disabled, frail or elderly patients;
- manning the shop that sells newspapers, soft drinks, sweets, and other small items that patients might need - the profits of the shop contribute to various hospital charities;
- providing a 'hospital car service' – volunteer drivers use their own cars (with expenses covered) to transport patients to and from hospital to enable them to keep appointments or receive treatment;
- raising funds to improve the hospital's facilities.

Activity

Find out if your local hospital is raising funds to improve the facilities. If so, produce a poster to describe the project.

9. a Why do hospitals have chaplains?
   b What is the purpose of a bereavement service?
   c Why does a hospital need volunteers?
   d For what activities may volunteers be used?

Complementary therapy

Complementary therapy (alternative medicine) provides treatment, or prevents illness, without using modern medicines. For most illnesses, it seems sensible for an ill person to seek advice from a doctor. If the advice or treatment does not help, the doctor or patient may then decide to try complementary therapy. There are many different therapies including those mentioned here.

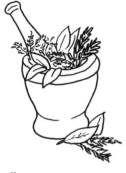

Herbalism
Medicines made from plants are used to prevent or treat disease.

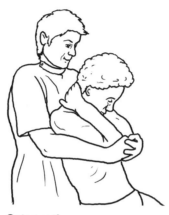

Osteopathy
Manipulation of muscles and joints.

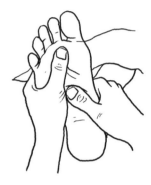

Reflexology
Different parts of the body are reflected in different areas of the feet, with massage applied to the appropriate area.

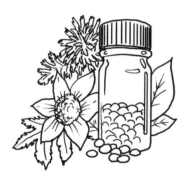

Homeopathy
An ailment is treated by minute doses of a substance that can, in larger doses, produce symptoms similar to those of the ailment itself.

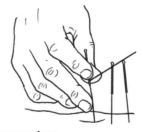

Acupuncture
Needles are inserted at specific points on the skin and, sometimes, rotated.

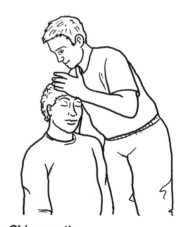

Chiropractic
Manipulation of the backbone to relieve pain.

Activity

Carry out a questionnaire to find out how many people in your local area have used complementary therapy and whether they think it worked to relieve their symptoms.
(➲ Questionnaire page 246.)

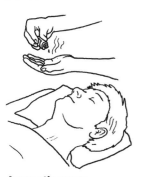

Aromatherapy
Aromatic oils such as lavender oil are inhaled, or absorbed through the skin during massage.

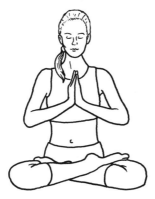

Yoga
Exercises to enhance breathing and muscle control.

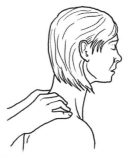

Shia-tsu
Similar to acupuncture but using finger pressure instead of needles.

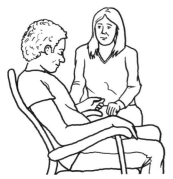

Hypnotherapy
A state of mild hypnosis is induced to relax the body and release the mind.

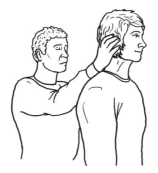

Alexander technique
Training to improve posture and movement when standing, walking, sitting or lying.

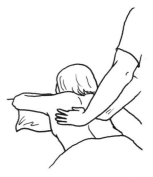

Healing by 'laying on of hands'
The healer's hands transmit healing influences to the troubled person or the damaged part.

10. a What is complementary therapy?
  b Name one therapy from pages 208-9 that involves:

manipulation,	posture,	hands,	fingers,
aromatic oils,	joints,	needles,	breathing,
plants,	hypnosis,	small doses,	feet.

Activity

Find out which health conditions each of the complementary therapies claims to treat.

Children's Trusts

A **Children's Trust** brings together (integrates) all the local services for children and young people in an area. Care workers from the different services work together to produce the best possible outcomes for children. This trust is intended for children and young people from birth to the age of 19 years to:

- be healthy;
- stay safe;
- enjoy and achieve;
- make a positive contribution;
- achieve economic well-being.

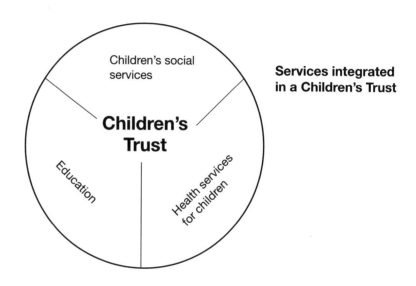

Services integrated in a Children's Trust

Sure Start

Sure Start is a programme to deliver the best start in life for every child. It brings together early education, child care, health and family support. It covers children until they reach the age of 14, and up to the age of 16 for those with special educational needs and disabilities.

Sure Start Children's Centres are places where children under five years' old and their families can receive integrated services and information. The services that are offered depend on local needs.

Activity

There is a separate Children's Commissioner for each part of the UK – England, Wales, Scotland and Northern Ireland – to promote the views and interests of children. Look at the website of the Children's Commissioner in your country to find out more about his/her job, and how he/she can be contacted. Compare your findings with the Children's Commissioner for another part of the UK.

1. **a** What does a Children's Trust do?
   b Name three services that are integrated in a Children's Trust.
   c What are the five aims of a Children's Trust?
   d **i** What is Sure Start,
   ii which children does it involve?
   e What happens in Sure Start Children's Centres?

Health services for children

Child health clinics (baby clinics)

These clinics are for the care of babies and pre-school children. Doctors, nurses and health visitors are there to:

- check the children's development;
- discuss any worries that parents might have;
- offer advice on matters such as feeding, hygiene and immunisation.

Immunisation The immunisation programme starts when a baby is two months old and continues throughout childhood. Vaccines are available to protect against a number of dangerous diseases common in childhood:

- diphtheria;
- pertussis (whooping cough);
- meningitis (Men C);
- rubella (German measles);
- tetanus;
- polio;
- measles;
- mumps;
- Hib vaccine (*Haemophilus influenzae type b*), gives protection against the bacterium which can cause pneumonia and meningitis;
- pneumococcal vaccine (pneumo jab) which gives protection against pneumonia, meningitis and blood infections.

School nurse

The school nurse is there for children, their parents, the staff and the well-being of the school. The nurse's duties include:

- carrying out health assessments on children when they enter the school, for example, height, weight, vision and hearing;
- providing first aid and nursing care when necessary;
- advising on the control of infectious diseases and infestations;
- providing a drop-in advice service in secondary schools;
- carrying out health promotion work, such as advising on healthy eating, sexual health and relationships, substance and alcohol abuse.

Dental health

Free dental care is available for children to check their teeth and gums at regular intervals, and to treat any problems. (➲ pages 114–115.)

Activity

Visit a child health clinic or family centre.
i   Describe the premises.
ii Explain what happens there.
iii Find out who is employed there and what they do.
iv Produce a leaflet that explains the work of the clinic and the people who work there.

2. a i Which professionals attend child health clinics,
     ii why are they there?
   b At what age does the vaccination programme start?
   c How many diseases are children vaccinated against?
   d What do school nurses do?
   e What dental care is available for children?

Family
support
groups.

Children
in care of
the local
authority.

Child
guidance
clinics.

Child
protection
teams.

Youth
work.

Youth
offending
services.

**Some of the Social
Services for Children**

Children's Social Services

Children's Social Services support children and families who have problems at home. They aim to protect the welfare of children by:

- supporting families with advice, information, practical support and counselling;
- supporting children with disabilities to allow them to lead lives that are as normal as possible;
- protecting children at risk of abuse or neglect;
- providing foster care, adoption services and residential accommodation for children who cannot live at home;
- providing support for young people who are leaving care to help them to live independently in the community;
- working with young people in trouble with the law.

How to get help

Families can approach Social Services directly to ask for support, or other professionals or members of the public may make Social Services aware of a problem. A social worker then visits the family and will need to speak to each of the family members individually to get an understanding of the situation. The social worker then assesses the situation and has a discussion with the family on what support would be useful, what is available, and to agree a way forward.

Criminal record checks

All adults who work with children must be positively vetted to ensure that they are appropriate people to work with children and vulnerable adults. They must therefore be checked by the CRB (Criminal Record Bureau) before they start work. This also applies to people who are going to work with vulnerable adults.

Activity

Invite a speaker from Social Services or a youth worker to talk to your group. Write a report on the talk. (➲ Writing a report page 242.)

3. a In what way do Children's Social Services support:
   i   families,
   ii children with disabilities,
   iii abused and neglected children,
   iv children who cannot live at home,
   v   young people leaving home,
   vi those in trouble with the law?
   b Name three ways that Social Services become aware of problems.
   c Who has to have a criminal record check before they start working with children?

Early Years Services

Early Years Services support the care and learning of pre-school children (those under five years' old). Education starts from birth as babies begin to learn about the people and world around them. It gathers pace as they start to play and attend pre-school groups. All three- and four-year-old children are guaranteed free, part-time early education in a pre-school group such as a nursery school or registered child-minding group or playgroup.

Pre-school groups

Pre-school groups offer care and early education to children under five years old, who attend on a part-time or full day basis. The groups are inspected regularly by **Ofsted** (Office of Standards in Education) – the organisation that inspects schools.

Day nurseries

At least half the staff in a day nursery must hold child care qualifications. The children are usually grouped according to age, with some nurseries taking babies at six weeks' old.

- **Private nurseries** are businesses that provide full day care for which fees are charged.
- **Community nurseries** provide full-day care on a not-for-profit basis for local families. Fees are generally lower than for private nurseries, and may be linked to parents' circumstances.
- **Local authority nurseries** cater mainly for families who need support. They usually open from 9 a.m. to 3 p.m., and some places may be free.
- **Workplace nurseries** are provided by employers for the children of their staff.

Registered childminders

Childminders work in their own homes looking after children whose parents are at work or studying. They are paid to provide a safe, caring environment that gives children opportunities for play and learning. Childminders do not need any qualifications, but they must be registered with Ofsted and complete an introductory childminding training course and a first aid course before they can become a childminder.

Playgroups

Playgroups offer opportunities for children to learn through play. They are run on a not-for-profit basis, and half the staff must hold qualifications in child care. Fees are charged to cover the running costs, although there may be some free part-time places.

Activity

Check that all the Early Years Services in your area are marked on your street map (➲ page 4).

---

4. **a** What is the purpose of the Early Years Services?
   b i What are pre-school groups,
      ii who inspects them?
   c Which Early Years Services:
      i may take six-week-old babies,
      ii take place in private homes,
      iii are not run for profit,
      iv places may be free? (Two answers for **iii** and **iv**.)
   d What conditions must be met before childminders can look after other people's children?

Working with children

There is a wide range of career opportunities in the areas of child care and early education. Some require qualifications, others are based on experience in bringing up children. There are also training courses that update knowledge and skills in the child care field.

Nursery nurses

Nursery nurses work with children from birth to around seven years of age. Their job is to care for and play with children, helping them to develop and learn. Jobs are available in day nurseries, in family centres and hospitals, as nannies in private homes, or to assist qualified teachers in infant classes.

Foster carers (foster parents)

Foster carers provide a family life for children who cannot live with their own parents. Foster care is often used to provide temporary care for children of all ages until their parents are able to look after them. Other children stay in long-term foster care or are adopted. Foster carers must attend a preparation course before they begin fostering a child.

SEN teaching

SEN (**Special educational needs**) teachers are responsible for children with emotional, behavioural or learning difficulties. **Qualified SEN teachers** and **learning support assistants** work in partnership to help the pupils reach the highest standards of personal achievement that they can. They work mainly in special classes in mainstream schools or in Special Schools.

Special Schools

Children in Special Schools need more individual care than is available in mainstream schools. Besides SEN teachers and learning support assistants they have:

- physiotherapists to train children with physical disabilities to make as full use as possible of their muscles;
- occupational therapists to help with training of skills for daily living;
- speech and language therapists to help those with speech and hearing difficulties.

Activity

Investigate a job working with children that you might like to do.

i   Describe the requirements of the job,

ii describe the skills needed for the job,

iii explain why the requirements for the job are necessary.

(➲ Writing a report page 242.)

5. **a** Describe the job of a nursery nurse.
   b Which care settings employ nursery nurses?
   c What do foster carers do?
   d Is foster care short or long term?
   e Do foster carers receive training?
   f What is an SEN teacher?
   g Describe five types of staff that work in Special Schools.

Youth workers

Youth workers help young people learn about themselves, other people and society through informal educational activities which combine enjoyment, challenge and learning. The young people are aged mainly between 13 and 19 years, although the range can extend from 11–25 years. Youth work takes place in many different settings and can be provided by local authorities or voluntary organisations. These groups include those that wear uniforms and also religious groups.

A youth worker can start without any qualifications if there is a commitment to a programme of training to achieve a qualification. There are two types of qualification:

- Youth Support Worker qualifications are NVQs and VRQs;
- Professional Youth Worker qualifications range from a Diploma in Youth Work to various Degrees in the subject – all the qualifications can be studied either part-time or full-time.

Young carers

Young carers are children who help look after a member of the family who is sick, disabled, has mental health problems or is misusing drugs or alcohol. The 2001 census showed that there are about 175 000 young carers in the UK, the average being 12 years old, 13 000 of whom give care for more than 50 hours a week. Their responsibilities can include cooking, cleaning, shopping, providing nursing and personal care and giving emotional support.

Barnardo's, the children's charity, states:

'Because young carers have adult responsibilities, they miss out on opportunities that other children have to learn and play. Many become chronically tired, struggle educationally and are often bullied for being 'odd'. They can become isolated, with no relief from the pressures at home, and no chance to enjoy a normal childhood. They are often afraid to ask for help as they fear letting the family down or being taken into care'.

Activity

a The charity for children, **Barnardo's**, runs projects that support young carers and keep families together. Find out what these projects are **(www.barnardos.org.uk).**

b Find out what support is offered by 'The Princess Royal Trust for Young Carers' **(www.youngcarers.net).**

c Give a talk of at least four minutes on 'Young carers and the problems they face'.
(➲ Media search page 245; ➲ Give a talk page 242.)

6. a What do youth workers do?
   b Does a youth worker need a qualification?
   c Describe two qualifications for youth workers.
   d i Who is a young carer,
      ii how many are there,
      iii what responsibilities do they have?
   e What do young carers miss out on?
   f What problems may they have?
   g Why may they be afraid to ask for help?

Access to care

Methods of referral

There are three ways in which people gain access to care services.

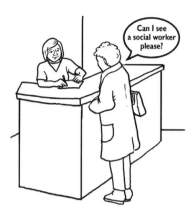

Self-referral occurs when a person telephones or visits a care centre for advice or treatment.

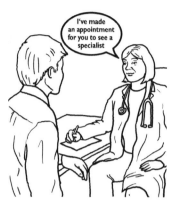

Professional referral occurs when a person is put in contact with a service by a care professional such as a doctor or social worker.

Methods of referral

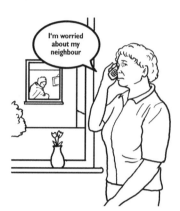

Third-party referral occurs when a relative, friend, neighbour, teacher or employer contacts a care service about someone else.

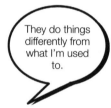

Barriers to obtaining care

There are a number of barriers that can prevent people from making use of the services they need. They include the following.

1. **Physical barriers** such as stairs, no lifts, doorways not wide enough for wheelchairs and no disabled toilets can all prevent access to services. This group also includes people who are too ill or disabled to leave their homes because of their physical condition.

2. **Psychological barriers** Some people do not seek help because they are afraid, embarrassed or ashamed. Perhaps they feel too shy to talk about their problems, or fear what they will be told. Others are too proud to be asking for help.

3. **Financial barriers** Not all NHS services are now free to everyone, for example some dental work, spectacles and some medicines have to be paid for. This is a barrier for those people who cannot afford to pay for the services they need, or for the cost of travel to get there. Social services are **means-tested** – this is the assessment of a person's finances to see if they can afford to pay some or all of the costs of the service. This can be a barrier to those who object to means-testing or fear that they cannot afford to pay.

4. **Geographical barriers** People in country areas may have more difficulty in obtaining health and care services, especially if they do not have their own transport. When specialist services are not available locally, the journey may be too long or cost too much.

5. **Cultural and religious barriers** People's personal views can prevent them from using the care services. For example, they may be too shy to talk about their problems, or prefer to discuss them only with their own sex or members of their own religion.

6. **Language barriers** Difficulties may arise when written instructions are not clearly explained, when there is a problem with deafness, or when the client cannot understand or read the language.

7. **Resource barriers** come about when:
   - there is a shortage of staff;
   - there is a lack of money to fund the service;
   - there is a lack of information about the service;
   - there is too high a demand for a particular service;
   - the person does not live in an area where the service is available – this is sometimes called the 'Postcode lottery'.

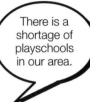

There is a shortage of playschools in our area.

There are no toilets nearby.

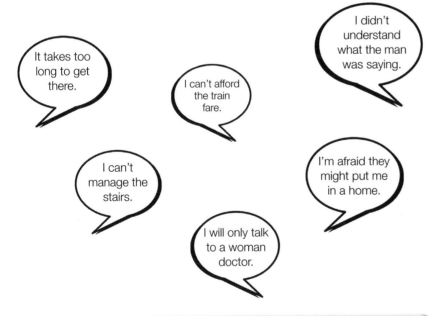

It takes too long to get there.

I can't afford the train fare.

I can't manage the stairs.

I will only talk to a woman doctor.

I didn't understand what the man was saying.

I'm afraid they might put me in a home.

The medicines cost too much.

It is too far to walk, and there aren't any buses.

1. Complete the chart by matching each of the seven barriers to obtaining care with two of the speech bubbles on pages 216 and 217.

Barrier	Example
1. Physical	**i** I can't manage the stairs **ii** ....

Activity

Use different examples to explain barriers to access of health and social care services. The examples could be from your own experiences, those of family or friends, or from reports in the media.

Partnership working

Partnership working is a way for individuals and agencies to work together to achieve a common aim. An **agency** is any organisation that is responsible for the delivery of services to individuals. **Multi-agency working** occurs when two or more agencies work together.

Partnership working is now commonplace in health and care settings. The partners can be:

- **individuals in a partnership** – they can be patients, clients, service users, carers, or family members.
- **agencies** – they can be:
  - public sector organisations;
  - private sector organisations;
  - voluntary organisations;
  - community organisations.

The purpose of working in partnership

When individuals and agencies work together to sort out a service user's problems they should:

- have a **holistic approach** – so that the whole person can be cared for by taking into account their physical, emotional, social, intellectual, cultural and religious needs;
- **identify common aims and objectives** – so that the individuals and agencies concerned with the problem are involved in the decision-making and planning;
- **coordinate the services** – link them together so that they can be delivered in a joined-up way;
- **reduce duplication** – which saves time and prevents irritation;
- **pool resources** – which saves money;
- **maximise expertise** – which makes best use of the special skills of everyone in the team;
- **ensure a consistent approach** – so that everyone knows what they are working towards and how to work together to achieve it.

Agencies

Social Services

Hospitals

Schools

Police

Health centres

Pre-school playgroups

Housing associations

Churches

Family centres

Probation service

---

1. **a** Explain the difference between 'partnership working' and 'multi-agency working'.
   b **i** What is an agency?
      ii Give some examples.
   c What is the advantage in partnership working of:
      i a holistic approach to a person's problems,
      ii identifying common aims,
      iii coordinating services,
      iv reducing duplication,
      v pooling resources,
      vi maximising expertise,
      vii a consistent approach.

Examples of working in partnership

Example 1: Pregnant school girl

The support provided to a pregnant teenager aims to help her care for herself and her baby, and to continue her education.

Doctor confirmed the pregnancy and arranged for antenatal care.

Sexual health clinic gave contraceptive advice to prevent another pregnancy.

Health visitor kept an eye on the family and advised on the baby's welfare.

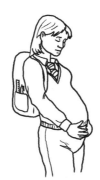

School has arranged for home tuition so that Trixie can keep up with her class work.

Midwife at the antenatal clinic arranged for the birth in hospital.

Trixie's mother accepted that Trixie would continue to live at home with her baby.

Example 2: Holistic approach to mental health

Helping people with mental illness achieve a healthier lifestyle involves a review of their physical health, their lifestyle and the home situation.

GP (doctor) for a health check-up to detect any underlying physical or emotional issues that need to be considered. Medication will be reviewed for unwanted side effects and to consider if it can be stopped.

Community psychiatric nurse to monitor Brad's mental health condition and ensure that he takes his medicine.

Dietitian for advice to encourage healthy eating.

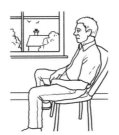

Brad had to give up work when he became mentally ill. Since his discharge from a psychiatric hospital he is hoping to regain his health and return to his old job.

Counsellor for a lifestyle assessment with questions about smoking, alcohol and any illegal drug use so that help and advice can be offered.

Occupational therapist who can suggest activities that prevent boredom and encourage socialisation and exercise.

Social worker to assess home conditions.

2. a In Example 1, describe:
   i   the individual and why she needs support,
   ii the partners who are providing the support.
  b Describe a holistic approach to mental illness.
  c In Example 2, describe:
   i   the individual and why he needs support,
   ii the partnership that supports him.

Activity

Clive is a single father with two children under five who is rapidly losing his sight due to an inherited genetic condition. He is very depressed and has been drinking a lot. Which professionals and organisations will be working in partnership to help Clive? Explain how each professional or organisation can benefit Clive and his family.

Example 3: Hospices

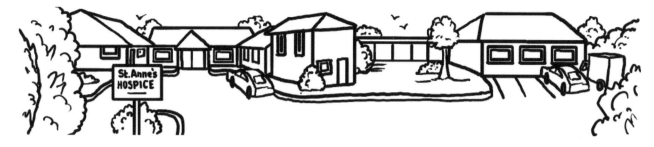

Hospices are for patients who are terminally ill. A **terminal illness** is one that will end in death. Hospices provide **palliative care** to improve the quality of life of patients and their families as they face the problems associated with terminal illness. Palliative care involves working in partnership, the partners being the patient, the relatives and all the professional and voluntary carers.

Palliative care provides:

- **skilled medical and nursing care** to relieve pain and other distressing symptoms;
- **emotional support** for those facing serious illness. Although death is inevitable, the focus in the hospice is on the quality of the life remaining, and on living life to the full;
- **support for the relatives and friends** of the patients;
- **carer support groups** with monthly meetings – the task of being the carer of a terminally ill patient can be very demanding and very isolating so, at group meetings, carers can share concerns and feelings;
- **a sitting service for patients** who are living at home, so that their carers can have a break or attend the monthly group meetings;
- **a bereavement service** to support bereaved relatives and friends, either one-to-one or in a group, with different religions catered for.

Hospices usually accept both day patients and in-patients. Visiting the hospice provides an outing for day patients and a break (respite) for their carers. Many in-patients stay for a week or two so that their carers at home can either have a break from caring or have a holiday. Patients who are too ill to be nursed at home can stay in the hospice long-term.

3. a What is:
  i a hospice,
  ii a terminal illness,
  iii palliative care?
b Who is a hospice for?
c Who is involved in palliative care?
d What does palliative care provide?
e Describe three groups who use hospices for varying amounts of time, and why.

Activities

1. Find out the whereabouts of your nearest hospice and what it offers, so that you can give a talk of at least four minutes.
2. Identify the needs of palliative care patients. Then identify how the different professionals meet these needs individually and together as a partnership.

Working in the health and social care sectors

There is a huge range of jobs to choose from in the health and social care sector. Some of these jobs need a qualification before beginning a career. Other jobs provide opportunities to develop skills through training. All applicants are required to undergo pre-employment checks (**vetting**) because they will later be in contact with vulnerable people. These include:

- **references** – character references from people who know you and/or employment references from current or previous employers.
- **a satisfactory interview.**
- **a CRB check** (Criminal Records Bureau ➲ page 212).
- **a PoCA check** (PoCA – Protection of Children Act) if the job involves working with children under the age of 18.
- **a PoVA check** (PoVA – Protection of Vulnerable Adults) if the job involves working in registered care homes or employment by domiciliary care agencies.

Personal attributes

People employed in the health and social care sectors are there to help the service users. Therefore, your appearance and personal qualities are important because these affect the way that clients and patients see you and react to you.

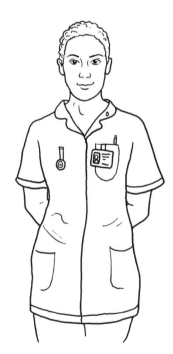

Facial expression A ready smile can help to make service users feel more at ease. Expressions of bad-temper, tiredness or indifference can easily upset them.

Empathy with others ➲ 7.

Ability to work with others: interpersonal skills (➲ page 62).

Registration with a professional body needs to be kept up-to-date.

Attitude This means the way a person thinks and behaves. A positive attitude is friendly and helpful. A negative attitude is hostile and resentful.

Confidence A confident manner encourages confidence in the service user.

Dress Looking clean, neat and appropriately dressed suggests hygienic and competent working practices.

Competence/qualifications need to be appropriate for the job and kept up-to-date.

Activity

If you were a patient or service user, place the personal attributes of carers listed above in the order of importance to you. Explain your decisions.

Workforce development

Induction

All new employees in health and social care, and those who are changing their roles and responsibilities, have to take part in an induction course. The aim is to enable health and social care workers to provide a high quality of care to service users, and to provide a basis for their own professional development.

Sector Skills Councils (SSC)

Sector Skills Councils for the different sectors of employment aim to develop a skilled UK workforce. The rules and regulations apply to England, Wales, Scotland and Northern Ireland although with some differences in each country.

- **Skills for Health** is the Sector Skills Council for the health sector and works to improve health and health care. It seeks to identify the future skills needed by the workforce and the education and training required.
- **Skills for Care & Development (SfC&D)** is the Sector Skills Council for social care, children and young people. Its purpose is to meet the UK's current and future social care needs for skilled and qualified workers.

National Minimum Standards

The National Minimum Standards set a minimum level of service for various parts of the care services. These guidelines make sure everyone understands what is expected and enables services to be measured against the same standards.

Terms and conditions

These are the rules of an agreement.

Activities

1. Find out:
   a which organisations are covered by the SfC&D.
   b which services are covered by the National Minimum Standards.
2. Explain the difference between a code of practice, policy, procedure and a charter. (➲ page 86.)

Chapter 9
The Impact of Diet on Health

This chapter covers:

- The dietary needs of individuals at different stages of life.

- The effects of unbalanced diets on the health of individuals.

- Specific dietary needs of patients/service users.

- The principles of food safety and hygiene.

Dietary needs of individuals

1. a What does the word 'diet' mean?
   b Why do people need food?
   c Name the five food groups in a balanced diet.
   d In a balanced diet, name:
      i three types of macro-nutrient,
      ii two types of micro-nutrient,
      iii two non-nutrients.
   e Why is water an essential part of the diet?
   f Explain the difference between DRVs and RDA.

Activities

1. Collect some examples of DRVs and RDAs from cereal packets.
2. i Produce a chart showing the RDAs for different nutrients for someone of your own age, and for someone over the age of 65.
   ii What changes take place in RDAs as people get older, and what stays the same?

Diet is the food and drink that a person regularly consumes to provide materials for growth, repair and replacement of body tissues, and for energy to keep the body alive and moving.

A balanced diet

A balanced diet is a healthy diet – one that contains all the five food groups in the appropriate amounts for the body to grow and function efficiently. The **five food groups** are:

- meat, fish, eggs and alternative non-animal protein foods;
- milk and other dairy foods;
- fruit and vegetables;
- foods containing fat and sugar;
- cereals, bread, rice, potatoes, maize and other staple foods.

Nutrients

Food and drink are composed of a mixture of nutrients and non-nutrients:

- **macro-nutrients** (macro = larger quantities);
  - **carbohydrates** – sugar and starch from plants,
  - **proteins** – from plant and animal sources,
  - **fats** – from plant and animal sources,
- **micro-nutrients** (micro = smaller quantities);
  - **vitamins** – A, B (complex), C, D, E and K,
  - **minerals** – calcium, sodium, iron, potassium and others,
- **non-nutrients**;
  - **fibre** (roughage) – material that cannot be digested,
  - **water** – about two-thirds of the body consists of water, which is essential to keep the body alive and healthy.

Dietary Reference Values (DRVs)

DRVs are estimates of the amount of energy (calories) and other nutrients needed by different groups of healthy people in the UK population. They are used by nutritionists as guidelines for assessing the diets of different groups of people. Although DRVs are given as daily intakes, people often eat quite different foods from one day to the next, and their appetites can change. In practice, the intakes of energy and nutrients need to be averaged over several days.

Recommended Daily Allowance (RDA)

An RDA is the suggested average daily intake of a nutrient that is needed in order to stay healthy. (page 229.)

Carbohydrates

Carbohydrates provide energy (calories) to keep the body alive and active.

They include:

- **sugars** – simple carbohydrates that are easy to digest and absorb;
- **starch** – complex carbohydrates that take longer to digest and absorb.

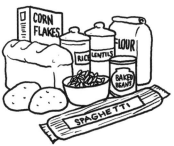

Starchy foods

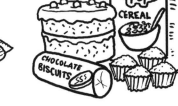

Foods rich in both starch and sugar

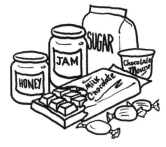

Sugary foods

Proteins

Protein foods are needed for growth and repair of the body. Protein is composed of tiny units called **amino acids**. The body requires 20 different types of amino acid. Nine of them are called **'essential amino acids'** because the body cannot make them, so they need to be present in the diet. The diet therefore should contain a variety of protein foods in order to ensure a supply of all the amino acids.

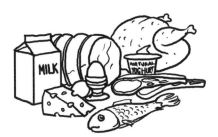

Animal proteins

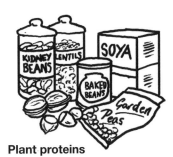

Plant proteins

2. a Name:
   i three groups of carbohydrate foods,
   ii two types of protein.
  b From each of the food groups shown above, choose the foods that you are likely to consume in a typical week and list them under five headings: starchy foods, sugary foods, starch and sugary foods animal protein, plant protein.

Activity

Choose at least 10 foods or drinks that you like. Find out whether each contains carbohydrates and proteins, and the proportion of each. Place your results in a table.

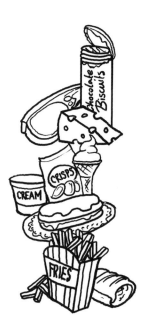

Foods containing fat

3. a Give two reasons for eating fat as part of the diet.

b Comparing saturated and unsaturated fats, which are:
  i usually solid at room temperature,
  ii usually liquid at room temperature,
  iii found in oily fish,
  iv found in animal foods,
  v found in mainly plant foods,
  vi may contain Omega 3.

c i What are trans fats,
  ii what are they made from and why,
  iii what are they used for,
  iv what is their disadvantage?

d Why is cholesterol essential in the body?

e Name the two sources of cholesterol.

f What is the danger of eating too much saturated fat?

g What are the risks of a high blood cholesterol level?

Fats and oils

Fats

Besides providing energy (calories), fat in the diet is needed to make the body's cells. Fats can be divided into two groups, saturated and unsaturated.

- **Saturated fat** is usually solid at room temperature. It comes mainly from animal foods such as meat, butter, cream, cheese, suet, lard, ghee and chocolate. A diet high in saturated fats is linked with heart disease.
- **Unsaturated fats** are usually liquid at room temperature and include mono-unsaturated and poly-unsaturated fats and fatty acids such as Omega-3. They come mainly from plants (olive oil, sunflower oil, nuts, seeds, avocados) and oily fish (salmon, mackerel, herrings, sardines, pilchards).

Trans fats

Trans fats are artificial fats. They are made from unsaturated fat which has been changed to give them a higher melting point and to extend their shelf life. They are popular for pastry, biscuits and muffins, but they increase the risk of coronary heart disease.

Cholesterol

Cholesterol is a natural part of food. It is found in all foods containing animal fats such as egg yolk, beef, chicken, cream, butter and cheese, and also in shrimps. It is essential in the body and has many functions:

- it is an important part of all cell walls in the body;
- it is a building block for making vitamin D in the skin;
- it is a building block for many hormones;
- it is used to make the fatty substance (myelin) that insulates nerve fibres and enables them to function efficiently.

Some cholesterol comes from food but most cholesterol is made in the body by the liver which can convert fat into cholesterol. If too much saturated fat is eaten, too much cholesterol may be produced. A high blood cholesterol level is a risk factor for coronary heart disease (➲ page 102).

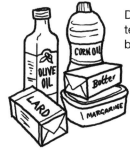

Depending on temperature, fats can be solid or liquid

Vitamins

Vitamins are essential substances that the body needs for growth and to be healthy and active. Only a very small quantity of each vitamin is required, and a balanced diet is likely to supply enough of them all. Taking too many vitamin supplements can be dangerous, especially the fat-soluble vitamins A and D because they can be stored in the body. This does not happen with vitamin C nor with most of the water-soluble B vitamins.

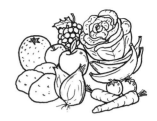

Fruit and vegetables are good sources of vitamins, minerals and fibre

	Important for	Good sources
Vitamin A	eyesight; growth; healthy skin	dairy foods, fish oils, carrots, green vegetables
B vitamins	Many functions. The B vitamins include B1, B2, B6, B12 and folic acid (⊃ page 229)	wholemeal bread, milk, cheese, liver, added to breakfast cereal, green leaves
Vitamin C	healthy gums; helps wounds to heal	fresh fruits and vegetables; the vitamin disappears during storage and when cooked
Vitamin D	healthy bones and teeth	margarine, butter, eggs, oily fish; made in skin when exposed to sunlight
Vitamin E	general health	most foods, and never in short supply
Vitamin K	blood clotting	made by bacteria in the large intestine and rarely in short supply

Minerals

Minerals are essential to the body in small amounts in order for it to work properly. Fifteen minerals are required including calcium, sodium, iron and potassium.

	Important for	Good sources
Calcium	strong bones and teeth	milk, cheese, yoghurt, white bread, green vegetables
Iron	production of red blood cells	red meat, eggs, green vegetables, bread, some breakfast cereals
Sodium	functioning of nerves and muscles	meat, poultry, fish, eggs; it is also part of the salt (sodium chloride) added to food
Potassium	functioning of nerves and muscles	most foods except fats and sugars.

4. Name a vitamin or mineral that is important for:
   i   the production of red blood cells,
   ii   blood clotting,
   iii helping wounds to heal,
   iv   nerves and muscles (two answers),
   v   healthy skin,
   vi   healthy gums,
   vii strong bones and teeth,
   viii eyesight.

Water

Water forms two-thirds of the body by weight and is present in all tissues. It is essential for life and needs to be kept at a more or less constant level. Therefore the water that is lost daily from the body in urine, sweat, breath and faeces needs to be replaced.

The amount of water an individual needs varies, and depends on:

- **the temperature of the body** – this rises when an individual is in a hot place or has a fever, and water is lost in sweat;
- **the weather** – people need more water in hot weather to replace that lost in sweat;
- **physical activity** – water is lost from the body in sweat and also by increased breathing;
- **diet** – the greater the content of water in the food that is eaten, the fewer drinks that are needed.

Dehydration occurs when more water is lost from the body than is taken in. The risk of serious dehydration is greatest in babies, older people and athletes. Obvious symptoms are thirst, dry lips and skin, small quantities of dark yellow urine, headaches, dizziness and exhaustion.

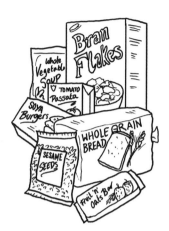

Foods containing fibre

2. **a i** About how much of the human body is water,
   ii where does this water come from,
   iii how is water lost from the body?
   b Why does the amount of water needed vary?
   c i When does dehydration occur,
   ii who is at greatest risk,
   iii what are its symptoms?
   d What is fibre?
   e Why is fibre important in the diet?
   f Which foods contain fibre?

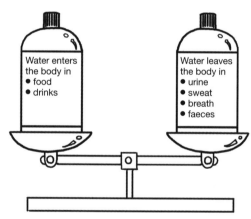

Water enters the body in
- food
- drinks

Water leaves the body in
- urine
- sweat
- breath
- faeces

Keeping water in the body in balance

Fibre

Fibre is the indigestible matter in food. It is important in the diet because it helps to keep food moving though the digestive system and helps to prevent constipation. Fibre is only found in foods that come from plants. Good sources include wholemeal bread, oats, pasta, peas, beans, lentils, nuts, fruit and vegetables.

Diet variations at different life stages

Babies

Breast milk is the ideal food for the first six months of life. It contains the right amounts of protein, sugar, vitamins, minerals and water needed for rapid growth and development. Breast milk does not contain iron as babies use the iron stored in the liver before birth. Bottle-fed babies are given formula milk, which is cows' milk that has been altered to make it more like human milk.

Weaning is the gradual changeover from a diet of milk to one based on a variety of food. It usually takes place at about six months of age as babies become able to digest starch. The baby now also needs foods that contain more vitamins, minerals and iron than are present in milk.

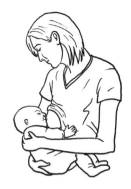

Breast milk is the natural food for babies

Age group	Males	Females
	kcal	kcal
Under 1 year	780	720
1 year	1200	1100
7–8 years	2000	1700
15–17 years	2800	2110
Adults	2500	1900
Pregnancy		2200
65+	2400	1900
75+	2150	1700

Recommended Daily Allowance (RDA) of calories (kcal) for different age groups

Childhood and adolescence

The need for foods containing energy increases as children become more active. The growing body also needs protein and all the vitamins and minerals. There is a marked increase in appetite during the growth spurt in early adolescence as larger quantities of all the nutrients are needed. Girls have a much higher need for iron than boys once menstruation starts.

Adults

Compared with adolescents, energy requirements are slightly lower for men. Although growth in height has ceased, the skin, hair and nails continue to grow, the red blood cells need constantly to be replaced, and the other tissues kept in good repair. Women who hope to become pregnant are advised to eat foods containing **folic acid** (a B vitamin) and, often, to take folic acid tablets to prevent birth defects such as spina bifida. During pregnancy and breastfeeding a little extra food is needed, especially foods containing calcium.

Older people

As people become less active, they need less food that supplies energy. But they still need a healthy diet with protein, vitamins, minerals and fibre. Because they may not feel as hungry as they used to, they may benefit from food that tempts the appetite.

6. **a** Why is breast milk the ideal food for young babies?
   b What is formula milk?
   c **i** What happens during weaning,
      ii Why is 6 months the usual age for weaning?
   d At what stage is there a marked increase in appetite?
   e When do girls have a higher need for iron?
   f Why do adults still need food for growth?
   g When do women need:
      i folic acid,
      ii extra calcium?

Activity

The Akhtar family includes Mr Abdullah Akhtar, his wife Shamina who is pregnant, their son Saeed who is 6 months old, their daughter Mysha who is 12 years old and Shamina's mother who is 74 years old. Produce an advice sheet for the family that gives suggestions for a balanced diet for each member of the family – which foods should they be eating to stay healthy, in what daily recommended amounts and why?

Socio-economic factors influencing the diet

The types of food and drink available

This will be influenced by the staple food of the area, for example wheat, rice, pasta, potatoes or maize. Also, living in the centre of a city or close to a supermarket allows greater variety in the diet than living in the country or depending on locally-produced food.

The level of physical activity

Exercise and hard physical work uses energy, which needs to be replaced by foods high in calories.

Medical conditions

These are discussed on pages 231–4.

Religious reasons

These are discussed on page 235.

Dieting

'Going on a diet' means making deliberate changes to the kinds or amount of food that is regularly eaten. People who diet in order to lose weight need to take in fewer energy foods.

Cultural reasons

People often eat the same kinds of food that their family and friends have always eaten.

Amount needed

The amount of food a person eats is influenced by:

- age (⮌ previous page);
- size – smaller people need less food than bigger people;
- gender – men usually eat more food than women of the same size;
- the environment – in cold weather or cold houses, people need more energy foods than in hot weather or over-heated buildings.

Personal preferences

People tend to stick with foods they know they like, and not to try different foods. Variety is also reduced by food fads (especially in children), bizarre health beliefs, and by being vegetarian.

The amount of money available for food

A low income results in a diet based on a limited range of cheaper foods, which may not include enough meat, fruit and vegetables.

Peer pressure

Diet can be influenced by peer pressure and the desire to conform to what others around you are eating.

The media

Advertising sweets and snacks during children's television programmes can encourage unhealthy eating and increase 'pester power'.

7. From the information given on this page, how many factors can you find that influence people's diet?

Activities

1. Find stories in the media that are about diet and the following factors: income; religion; geographical locations (e.g. inner city diets and rural diets) and personal preference. Produce a poster using pictures and quotes from the media stories to show socio-economic influences on diet.
2. Give a four minute talk on 'You are what you eat'.

The effects of unbalanced diets on health

An **unbalanced diet** contains too much or too little of one or more nutrients. For example, too much fat or salt, or too little protein, vitamin A or iron. This upsets the chemical balance in the body and results in malnutrition. **Malnutrition** is a condition caused by insufficient food, too much food or an unbalanced diet. Malnutrition therefore includes both over-nutrition and under-nutrition.

Over-nutrition

Over-nutrition is the excessive intake of energy foods – those containing fat and carbohydrates (sugar and starch). When a person eats more of these foods than are needed to supply energy, the excess becomes stored as body fat. That person then becomes overweight or obese. (➲ BMI page 149.) Over-nutrition is an increasing problem in the UK and other developed countries.

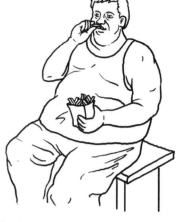

Fat is stored under the skin of the chest, abdomen and bottom, and around the heart, kidneys and other organs in the abdomen.

Obesity

Obesity is caused by taking in more energy foods than the body needs. It results from:

- the enjoyment of eating too much;
- the compulsion to eat too much;
- eating when bored or anxious;
- failing to take enough exercise.

Obesity is associated with many illnesses and is directly related to lower life expectancy. Medical conditions resulting from obesity are:

- coronary heart disease (➲ page 102);
- Type 2 diabetes (➲ page 136);
- osteo-arthritis in hips and knees (➲ page 95).

Bulimia nervosa

Bulimia is compulsive over-eating. People with this condition are worried about putting on weight, but cannot control their eating. Typically, a binge on food is followed by self-induced vomiting or excessive use of laxatives. It can occur at any age but often starts in the teens, with women more likely to be affected than men. It may accompany anorexia nervosa (➲ page 232).

---

1. a What is an unbalanced diet?
  b Give three causes of malnutrition.
  c What is over-nutrition?
  d How is excess food stored in the body?
  e Where is fat stored in the body?
  f i What causes obesity,
    ii what does it result from,
    iii what medical conditions are linked with it?
  g i What is bulimia,
    ii what follows the over-eating,
    iii who are more likely to be affected,
    iv why does it occur?

Activities

1. Identify two medical conditions related to unbalanced diets.
2. Describe how these diets result in the development of the medical condition.

Under-nutrition

Under-nutrition occurs when the diet is short of one or more of the nutrients in food. It can be due to:

- poverty – lack of money to buy enough food;
- an unbalanced diet;
- an inability to feed oneself;
- a defect in the body's ability to absorb the food.

Starvation The body can usually cope with under-nourishment for a short time without lasting ill-effects. Long-term it results in severe under-nourishment and starvation. Starvation (protein-energy malnutrition) is rare in developed countries like the UK, but common in less developed parts of the world. It causes:

- **marasmus** in infants, due mainly to a deficiency of energy;
- **kwashiorkor** in children, due mainly to protein deficiency.

Specific nutrient deficiency

The shortage or absence of one nutrient in the diet affects the normal activity of the body. For example:

- **deficiency of vitamin A** causes blindness in about half a million children in a year world wide. Night blindness is an early symptom.
- **deficiency of B1** (thiamine) causes beriberi. This disorder of the heart and nervous system is widespread in communities that have a diet based on polished rice. When rice is polished, the seed coat which is rich in thiamine is removed.
- **deficiency of vitamin C** (ascorbic acid) causes scurvy. The first sign is swollen bleeding gums which may be followed by easy bruising and anaemia.
- **deficiency of vitamin D** causes rickets in children and osteomalacia in adults (muscular weakness, bone pain and a tendency to fracture).
- **deficiency of iron** causes anaemia.

Anorexia nervosa

Anorexia is a serious emotional illness in which the patient either refuses food or eats under protest and then secretly vomits. It most often occurs in teenage girls who think that they are too fat even though they may be thin. This illness leads to such severe loss of weight that the bones stick out and the periods stop. The patient may become too weak to stand and needs hospital care and skilled counselling.

2. **a** **i** What is under-nutrition?
   ii Give four causes.
   b Describe two conditions caused by starvation.
   c What is a specific nutrient deficiency?
   d Which nutrient is deficient in cases of:
   i rickets,
   ii scurvy,
   iii beriberi,
   iv some forms of blindness,
   v some forms of anaemia?
   e **i** Who are most at risk of anorexia, and why?
   ii what are the effects of the illness?

Activity

Find information about kwashiorkor (pronounced quosh-ee-or-kor) and marasmus. Summarise the information in a chart to show the differences between these two diseases of malnutrition, and how to treat them.

Specific dietary needs

Disease of the arteries

A healthy diet is one that is low in saturated fat, sugar, salt and contains at least five portions of fruit and vegetables a day. Saturated fat should be avoided as it encourages the body to make cholesterol. This can build up on artery walls and lead to coronary heart disease (➲ page 102).

Foods that help to reduce the risk of coronary heart disease are:

- oily fish such as salmon and sardines;
- many fruits, vegetables and cereals contain antioxidants that prevent saturated fats from being changed into cholesterol;
- beans, peas, lentils, nuts and oats contain soluble fibre that helps to lower the cholesterol level.

Obesity

The most successful weight loss programmes usually include:

- **taking in fewer calories** by choosing foods low in calories and eating smaller portions;
- **taking more exercise** as being active uses up the calories contained in the food.

Diabetes

Although there are different treatments for Type 1 and Type 2 diabetes, the dietary advice is the same for both types.

- Regular balanced meals are most important.
- The diet must be low in sugar and fat, especially saturated fat.
- The diet must be low in salt.
- Each meal should contain:
  — some starchy food such as bread, rice, pasta or potatoes;
  — a normal amount of protein;
  — high-fibre foods (wholemeal bread, fruit and vegetables). The presence of fibre helps to control blood sugar levels by slowing the absorption of sugar from the gut.
- There is no need for special diabetic foods. They are expensive and unnecessary, and are no substitute for a healthy diet.

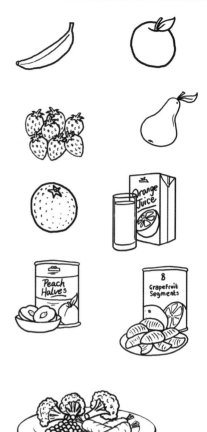

3 portions

3 portions

Examples of portions of fruits and vegetables

1. **a** Describe a healthy diet.
   b Describe a portion of strawberries, peaches, grapefruit, fruit juice, broccoli and carrots.
   c What is the effect on cholesterol of:
      i fruit, vegetables and cereals,
      ii beans, peas and lentils?
   d Name three things that are part of a weight loss programme.
   e Give five pieces of advice recommended for a diabetic diet.

Activity

Find out about coeliac disease and phenylketonuria – two conditions with specific dietary needs.
i Produce a two-day dietary plan for a patient with each disease – breakfast, lunch, dinner, snacks and beverages.
ii Identify what a balanced diet for each patient will need to include.

Lactose intolerance

This is the inability to digest lactose (milk sugar). Lactose is found in milk from mammals (cows, goats, sheep) and in products made from milk (cream, cheese, yoghurt). It is also added to many foods such as ice cream, salad cream, biscuits, chocolate, sweets, cakes and peanut butter. The condition can be avoided by omitting foods that contain lactose from the diet. People with mild lactose intolerance often find that they can eat cheese because it contains much less lactose than milk.

Food allergies

A number of foods are known to cause allergies, for example milk, egg, wheat, soya, seafood, fruit and peanuts. Allergic reactions affect people in different ways and produce many different symptoms. An allergic reaction does not happen the first time the food is eaten because the body needs to develop sensitivity to that food before it can become allergic. The best way to prevent an allergic reaction is to avoid the food that causes the condition.

Food and behaviour

Research into what people eat shows that it can affect how they think and behave. The following are some examples.

- Individuals eating an unhealthy diet were more likely to commit serious offences compared with those whose diet was more healthy.
- When inmates at a juvenile detention centre had more fruit and vegetables in their diet and the intake of sugar and soft drinks reduced, the number of disciplinary incidents was reduced by half.
- Adolescents who cannot be persuaded to eat a healthy diet show more control over their mood swings and behaviour when given appropriate vitamin and mineral supplements.
- Children who are energetic and funny when they eat fresh food can become disrupting, tormenting and miserable when they are fed on sweets, crisps, fizzy drinks and processed food.

2. **a** What is lactose intolerance?
   b Why do people with lactose intolerance need to take care before eating biscuits?
   c Give some examples of foods known to cause allergies.
   d Why does an allergic reaction not occur the first time a food is eaten?
   e What caused a reduction of disciplinary offences in a juvenile detention centre?
   f Give two suggestions for reducing mood swings.

Activity

Use the internet to find research papers on the effect of diet on behaviour. Select two examples and summarise the information from each.

Religion and culture

The culture of a country influences the diet of the people who live there. The diet may also be affected by the rules of their religion.

Christians There are no dietary restrictions, so all types of food can be eaten, although some Christians may prefer to eat fish on Fridays, or fast on Fridays or during Lent for spiritual reasons.

Jews have strict rules about their diet: pork and seafood are not allowed and dairy and meat foods may not be mixed together. Kosher food is prepared in accordance with Jewish dietary laws.

Muslims No pork is allowed and other meat should be prepared by the halal method. No alcohol is allowed.

Buddhists are vegetarian.

Hindus Most Hindus are strict vegetarians. Hindus who normally eat meat will not eat anything that contains beef or beef products, because the cow is a sacred animal.

Sikhs Most Sikhs are vegetarian and do not eat eggs or fish or any foods made from them. Sikhs are not allowed to consume alcohol as they need to be alert at all times.

Vegetarians do not eat meat or fish. Their diet provides all the necessary amino acids from the proteins in grains, beans and nuts and other plant foods. Strict vegetarians (**vegans**) do not eat any food derived from animals such as fish, dairy foods, eggs or honey. Their diet can then be low in calcium, iron, vitamin B_{12} and vitamin D. These can be provided by taking dietary supplements.

Dietitians

Registered dietitians (RDs) are experts in diet and nutrition, so they can provide advice on all aspects of eating and diet, including special diets for medical conditions. The title 'dietitian' is protected by the Health Professionals Council (HPC). This means that someone can't call themselves a dietitian unless they are suitably qualified and registered with the HPC. Registered dietitians are regulated by the HPC. The professional association for dietitians is the British Dietetic Association.

3. **a** When planning menus for patients, which religious group:
   i does not eat beef,
   ii would not want bacon and cheese flan,
   iii do not eat pork products,
   iv might prefer fish on a Friday?
   b Name the religious groups that:
   i do not consume alcohol,
   ii are vegetarian.
   c Explain the difference between a vegetarian and a vegan.
   d What supplements are vegans advised to take and why?

Activity

Use the internet to find out how to become a dietitian:
i the qualifications needed to start training,
ii the qualifications received when training is complete,
iii the variety of jobs open to a trained dietitian.

Food safety and hygiene

Food hygiene means keeping food clean and safe to eat. Occasionally food becomes contaminated by chemicals used in its production or manufacture. Rarely, it is contaminated by unwanted objects such as a piece of glass or a dead fly. In nearly all cases, food that causes illness has been contaminated by food-poisoning bacteria.

Food poisoning

Food poisoning is caused when food or drink becomes contaminated with bacteria or the toxins (poisons) that they produce. Bacteria thrive in warm, moist foods, particularly those containing protein, for example meat and fish, eggs and milk. In these conditions, bacteria multiply by repeatedly dividing in two, and large numbers can be built up very quickly. They cause illness when:

- large numbers of bacteria are eaten;
- the food contains toxins produced by some types of bacteria;
- the food has been contaminated by bacterial spores. Some bacteria produce spores that can survive for a long time in dust and dirt. The spores are not killed by cooking and, if the food is cooled slowly or kept warm before eating, the spores germinate, multiply and produce very heat-resistant toxins (poisons) which are not destroyed by re-heating.

Symptoms

The typical symptoms of food-poisoning (gastro-enteritis) are:

- abdominal pain;
- vomiting;
- diarrhoea.

The severity of the illness varies considerably depending on:

- the type of food-poisoning bacteria involved;
- the amount of poisoned food eaten;
- the health of the individual – people who are very young, old or ill are most at risk of illness.

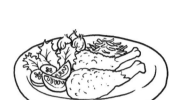

It is hard to tell if food is contaminated by food poisoning because the look, taste and smell may not be affected.

1. **a** What is food hygiene?
   b What are nearly all cases of illness caused by food due to?
   c What causes food poisoning?
   d In what conditions do food-poisoning bacteria thrive and multiply?
   e When do food-poisoning bacteria cause illness:
      i what are the symptoms,
      ii why does the severity of the illness vary?

Food-poisoning bacteria

Salmonella species
There are over 200 different types of salmonella. They are usually found in poultry, eggs, unprocessed milk and in meat and water. One species of salmonella causes typhoid.

E. coli are normally found in the intestines of animals and humans. One uncommon type which can cause serious illness is E. coli 157. This has been found in raw and undercooked meats, unpasteurised milk and dairy products, raw vegetables and unpasteurised apple juice.

Campylobacter species are found in the intestines of wild birds, pets, poultry and untreated water or milk.

Staphylococcus aureus commonly lives on the skin of the hands and in the noses of healthy and unhealthy people.

Bacillus cereus
Spores of bacillus cereus are found in soil and dust. It is frequently found in rice dishes that have not been cooled quickly after cooking, and then kept cold.

Clostridium perfringens produces spores that survive in dust and dirt.

Bacteria that cause food poisoning

Food Standards Agency (FSA)

The Food Standards Agency is an independent Government department set up by an Act of Parliament in 2000. It aims to make sure that food is safe to eat by giving advice and information to the public and Government on:

- food safety from farm to fork;
- nutrition and diet;
- advice on food allergy;
- hygiene and information about food poisoning;
- effective food enforcement and monitoring.

The FSA's strategic plan 2005–10 has as its key aims:

- to continue to reduce food-borne illness;
- to reduce further the risks to consumers from chemical contamination including radiological contamination of food;
- to make it easier for all consumers to choose a healthy diet, and thereby improve quality of life by reducing diet-related disease;
- to enable consumers to make informed choices.

2. **a** Which bacteria:
   i are found in intestines,
   ii live on the skin,
   iii can cause typhoid,
   iv produce spores,
   v are found in dust and dirt,
   vi can occur in cold rice,
   vii can occur in water,
   viii can occur in milk.
   b What are the key aims of the Food Standards Agency?

Activity

Carry out a media search for new items about food-poisoning cases for a display on this subject.

Preventing food poisoning

The essential rules to prevent food poisoning are:

- wash your hands thoroughly before handling food;
- keep food clean to prevent contamination;
- keep food cold to prevent bacteria from multiplying;
- cook food thoroughly to kill any bacteria.

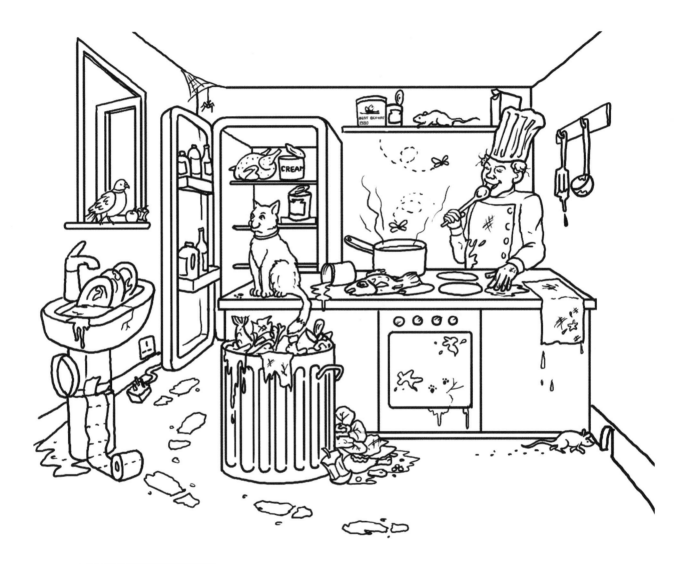

3. What are the four essential rules to prevent food poisoning?

Activities

1. In the picture above, how many unsafe practices can you spot that could give rise to food poisoning? Can you find at least 20?
2. Watch the video 'Bacteria Bite Business' that is available from the Food Standards Agency website as it covers the four Cs of good food hygiene – Cleaning, Cooking, Chilling and Cross-contamination. Discuss the video and its usefulness in helping to reduce cases of food poisoning.

Legislation, regulations and codes of practice

Food Safety Act 1990

Anyone who handles food, or cleans equipment that comes into contact with food, or whose actions could affect its safety must follow the regulations in this Act. In health and safety settings:

- food handlers must protect food against contamination that could cause a health hazard;
- food handlers must receive adequate training and supervision;
- the owners of the businesses are responsible for ensuring that the hygiene standards that are laid down in the regulations are maintained on their premises;
- premises that cause imminent risk to health can be closed down.

The Food Safety (General Food Hygiene) Regulations 1995

The aim of these regulations is to ensure common food hygiene rules across the European Community (EC).

Food Safety (Temperature Control) Regulations 1995

- Food which is likely to support the growth of food-poisoning microbes must not be kept above 8°C.
- Food which has been cooked or re-heated must be kept at or above 63°C.

Hazard Analysis Critical Control Point (HACCP)

This is an international management system to identify hazards in food production and preparation to ensure that food is safe for human consumption.

Food Law Code of Practice

The Food Law Code of Practice is published by the Food Standards Agency. It sets out instructions for local authorities on how to comply with food legislation.

---

4. a i Who is the Food Safety Act 1990 intended for?
  ii Describe four ways in which the regulations could affect a Residential Care Home.
  b What regulations affect the UK and all other countries in the EC?
  c Which types of food must be:
   i kept at or above 63°C,
   ii not kept above 8°C?

Chapter 10
Study Skills

This chapter covers:

- Building a portfolio.
- Answering questions.
- Making notes.
- Writing a report.
- Giving a talk.
- Group discussions.
- Role play.
- Planning an activity.
- Media searches.
- Questionnaires.

Study skills

Study skills are the skills that enable you to learn more easily and to produce a higher standard of work. This book provides opportunities for you to develop the skills for your portfolio when you:

- answer written questions;
- make notes;
- write a report;
- give a talk;
- take part in group discussions;
- role play;
- carry out an internet search.

Building a portfolio

Your portfolio is a personal record of work done during the course. It provides evidence of the topics studied and the progress that you have made. It also enables you to demonstrate knowledge and understanding of the subject and skills in literacy, numeracy and IT.

Presentation When complete the portfolio needs to be:

- well presented – neat, orderly, unfussy, arranged in a logical order and with a contents list;
- legible – so that it can be easily read;
- accurate;
- grammatically correct (correct spelling and punctuation).

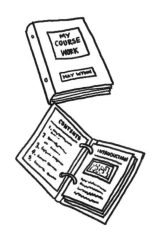

Answering questions

Most pages in this textbook have a bank of questions. This is an immediate check on what has been learned. The answers should be hand-written as this gives practice in writing neatly and clearly – skills that are valued by employers.

When answering a question, **one-word answers are no use**. They will mean nothing to you when you look at your work again, nor to anyone else who assesses your work.

Points to note:

- Always answer a question with a complete sentence.
- Start a sentence with a capital letter and finish it with a full stop.
- Remember that writing must be legible, that is, clear enough to be read easily.
- Check your spelling and punctuation.
- Ask your tutor to check samples of your work to see if it is satisfactory.

Question
What is communication?

Answer
Communication is the exchange of information.

Making notes

Notes do not need to be written in sentences, but they will only be useful if they are:

- clear;
- concise;
- easy to understand.

Writing a report

A report is a detailed description of a particular event. Everything needs be clearly explained because the reader cannot be expected to know anything about the event. Reports:

- should have a title;
- should start off with an introduction to explain why the report is being written;
- should be written in paragraphs, or in sections with headings;
- may include drawings, photographs or any other helpful information;
- have a concluding paragraph that sums up the report.

Giving a talk

Preparation

- Decide on the topic of your talk.
- Find out how long the talk should last.
- Make notes of the important points you wish to mention.
- Decide if you are happy for your audience to ask questions.
- Practise giving your talk, and time yourself.
- Adjust your talk to fit into the required time.

When giving your talk

- First of all, explain what your talk is about.
- Speak directly to the audience.
- Speak clearly, don't mumble, don't rush and don't ramble.
- Use words and expressions that everyone can understand.
- Use audiovisual aids (photographs, leaflets, flip charts, video clips, music, items of interest) that help to explain the purpose of your talk.
- Conclude with a brief summary by reminding your audience of the main points.
- Ask if there are any questions (if appropriate).
- Thank the audience for listening.

When giving a talk

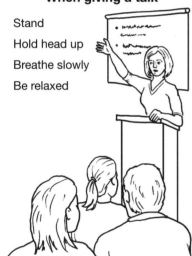

Stand
Hold head up
Breathe slowly
Be relaxed

Group discussions

Planning a discussion

Decide:

- the title of the discussion;
- the time allowed for the discussion;
- the maximum time allowed for each speaker;
- who will 'chair' the discussion, or be in charge;
- who will open the discussion;
- the order in which the rest of the group will speak;
- when questions can be invited;
- who will sum up the discussion;
- if a video recording or audio tape-recording is to be made.

Ground rules

Ground rules need to be set before a group discussion takes place. For example:

- everyone is expected to contribute to the discussion;
- no-one speaks for more than a set length of time (and how to police this);
- everyone is allowed to put a point of view;
- no-one interrupts another speaker;
- there is no personal criticism of others in the group, though constructive criticism is to be encouraged;
- language that could offend is not used;
- hostile body language or tone of voice is avoided.

Report on the discussion

This can be a personal account presented as a written report or as an analysis of a video or audio recording. For example, a report should have:

- the title of the discussion;
- your personal contribution to the discussion;
- points made by the different speakers;
- any conclusions reached by the group;
- any unresolved disagreements;
- whether the ground rules were followed.

Self-appraisal

Good communication is central to working in health and social care and involves a number of skills. During the discussion, how would you rate or comment on your skill in:

- listening;
- understanding;
- asking questions;
- manner of speaking;
- using body language?

Role play

Role play involves a situation in which actors express different points of view or types of behaviour. Taking part in role play helps:

- in researching and presenting other points of view;
- to develop confidence in speaking out;
- to develop the skill of listening to others and practising other communication skills;
- to experience other people's points of view and accept that they can be different from your own;
- in reinforcing the course work.

Planning role play

Decide:

- the size of the role play group(s);
- the situation to be acted out;
- who is to play which role – everyone is expected to take part in role play at some stage, even if in only a small way – it is surprising how much even the most anxious students can enjoy the experience once they have played a role;
- how much time is to be allowed for the actors to think about, or discuss, their role;
- if a video or audio recording is to be made.

Ground rules

Before role play takes place, ground rules need to be set in advance. For example:

- all actors are allowed to act out their roles in their own ways;
- no-one watching may interrupt the actors;
- personal comments are not allowed.

Assessment of the role play

- Were the ground rules followed?
- What skills were demonstrated?
- In what ways did the role play reinforce the course work?

Self-assessment

What did you learn from the role play – taking part, listening, understanding different points of view and coping with emotional situations?

Planning an activity

When planning an activity:

- think clearly about what it is that you want to do;
- where you are going to do it;
- how you are going to do it;
- what equipment is needed;
- how much time is required to complete the activity.

Media search

A media search is a search for information from books, newspapers, journals, magazines or the internet.

Points to note:

- A search is more valuable if it is organised and the details are recorded.
- Quality of information is more important than quantity.
- The skill in making a media search is in deciding what is to be included and what excluded.
- Merely printing out pages from the internet is **not** a media search – you may just get a random collection of unrelated facts.

Stages of a search

1. **Find a good title for your search** – this will help guide you to the information you are looking for.

2. **How much time do you have available** for the search – how much time is it reasonable to spend?

3. **Where should you search?** Find information from:
   - people, for example, witnesses, experts, etc.;
   - written sources such as books, newspapers, journals, magazines – all found in public libraries, often with helpful librarians;
   - recorded sources, for example, tapes, music, CD, DVDs;
   - the internet.

4. **For each source of information**, make a note of where the information comes from and the date that you accessed it.
   - For a **book**, record:
     - the title;
     - the publisher;
     - publication date;
     - the author;
     - the page number/s.
   - For a **newspaper or magazine article**, record:
     - the title of the newspaper or magazine;
     - the date of issue;
     - the author of the article (if known).
   - For the **internet**, record:
     - the name of the organisation;
     - its web address;
     - the title of the page that contained the information.

Questionnaires

A questionnaire is a type of survey that uses a list of questions to obtain facts or opinions from a number of people.

- Decide what information is required.
- Design the questions.
- Design a suitable form to record the answers.
- Select a sample of people to be questioned.
- Ask the questions and record the answers.
- Analyse the answers.
- Draw your conclusions and present them in an appropriate way.

Glossary

Abscess   a collection of pus in a cavity surrounded by inflamed tissue

Abuse   the deliberate ill-treatment of other people. Abuse can be: physical, emotional, neglect, sexual, or financial

Acne   a rash with spots (painful red nodules and 'blackheads') mostly on the face; most common in adolescence

Acute   lasting a short time. *See* **Chronic**

Ageing   a natural process of gradual change that proceeds throughout adulthood and results in reduced function

Agency   any organisation responsible for the delivery of services to individuals

Allergy   an immune reaction by the body to a particular substance such as dust mites, pollen, pets and nuts

Anaemia   a shortage of haemoglobin in the blood

Anatomy   the structure of the body and its various parts

Angina   a characteristic pain in the centre of the chest due to heart disease

Anti-social behaviour   behaviour that is harmful or annoying to others. *See* **Pro-social behaviour**

Artery   carries blood away from the heart

Asthma   a lung condition with wheezing, shortness of breath and coughing

Atheroma   thickening of the arteries. *See* **Plaque**

Bacteria (singular, bacterium)   a group of microbes that can cause disease

Balanced diet   a diet that contains all five food groups in the appropriate amounts for the body to grow and function efficiently

Bedsores   *See* **Pressure sores**

Beliefs   religious or non-religious thoughts, feelings, attitudes and values that an individual believes to be true

Blindness   the absence of useful sight. Most blind people have some awareness of light

Blood pressure (BP)   the pressure of blood in a main artery

Blood vessels   tubes through which blood flows as it circulates around the body. *See* **Artery**, **Vein**, **Capillary**

Body language   communication by movements or position of the body

Boredom   uninterested in anything due to being mentally under-occupied

Bruise   discoloured area that follows trauma to the body with bleeding under the skin

Bullying   when one or more people repeatedly intimidate and persecute a weaker person

Capillary   a very small blood vessel that links arteries to veins. Capillaries have very thin walls so substances such as oxygen, carbon dioxide and food pass through the walls

Cardiac arrest   the heart stops beating properly and no longer circulates blood around the body

Care needs   the young, old, sick, disabled and distressed need care; medical, nursing, social and personal

Care professionals   specially-trained people who have gained the relevant qualifications (e.g., doctors, nurses, social workers)

Care values   beliefs about the correct way to treat people receiving care

Care value base   a set of values and principles for care workers

Care workers/Carers   people who look after those who cannot look after themselves (e.g., support workers, care assistants and home carers)

Cell   a tiny unit of living matter

Census   an official count of the population in an area

Charter   a document that sets out the service that users can expect to receive

Cholesterol   a fatty chemical in blood and tissues of animals. It is an essential part of a healthy body

Chronic   lasting a long time. *See* **Acute**

Circulation   Blood continuously circulates from the heart to the lungs to collect oxygen, and then back to the heart to be pumped to all the parts of the body before returning to the heart again.

Code of practice   guidelines for how people should behave and carry out duties

Communication   the exchange of information (facts, feelings, news, etc.) between individuals, groups or organisations

Communication cycle   the pathway of a message passing from person to person

Conception   occurs when an egg is fertilised

Confidentiality   keeping information secret

Convulsions   unnatural jerking movements

Creative activities   these aim to produce something original. *See* **Therapeutic activities**

Culture   the way of life of a group of people including their customs and values

CV (Curriculum vitae)   an outline of a person's educational and professional history

Cystitis   inflammation of the bladder

Deafness   some loss of hearing, seldom total

Delirium   mental confusion

Dermatitis   *See* **Eczema**

Dermis   the inner layer of skin. *See* **Epidermis**

Dietitian   a person who has completed a BSc Honours degree in Nutrition and/or Dietetics

Disability   difficulty or inability to carry out normal everyday activities because of mental or physical problems

Disclosure   to reveal information

Discrimination   the different, often unfair, treatment of a person or group of people

Diversity   the way that individual people are different from each other in a society

Drug addiction   uncontrolled craving for drugs due to physical and psychological dependence

DVT (Deep Vein Thrombosis)   a blood clot in a vein, usually in the calf or thigh

Eczema (Dermatitis)   a dry, red, itchy rash

Embryo   a developing baby during the first seven weeks after conception. *See* **Fetus**

Empathy   feeling yourself in someone else's situation. *See* **Sympathy**

Encephalitis   inflammation of brain tissue

Epidermis   the outer layer of skin. *See* **Dermis**

Equality   giving equal treatment to people in similar situations so that the same opportunities exist for everyone

Equality of opportunity   equal rights to employment, medical treatment and other services

Ethnic group (ethnicity)   people with the same racial origins and cultural traditions

Excretion   the removal of waste products from the body

Family   a group of individuals who live together and are related by blood, marriage or adoption

Fetus   a baby from 7 weeks until birth

Fever   a rise in body temperature above normal

Fibre   indigestible matter in food; not absorbed; important for the normal function of the colon

Gender (sex)   male or female

Gender identity   the gender to which a person feels he or she belongs

Gender roles   the attitudes and behaviours considered more appropriate for one gender or the other within a culture

Germs   micro-organisms (microbes), mainly bacteria and viruses that cause disease

Growth and development   growth is an increase in size; development refers to an increase in abilities (what a person is able to do)

Haemoglobin   the red substance in red blood cells that carries oxygen

Harassment   persistent offensive or intimidating behaviour

Hazard   anything that can cause harm. *See* **Risk**

Health   'a state of complete physical, mental and social well-being and not merely the absence of disease and infirmity' (WHO)

Health and Social Care   the study of the care services

Heart attack   the death of a part of the heart muscle

Heart failure   (a misleading term) the heart has not failed to work; it is not pumping as strongly as it should

Holistic (in medicine)   considering a patient as a whole person both physically and psychologically

Hospice   a place for patients with terminal illness and their families

Hygiene   concerned with cleanliness and the prevention of the spread of infectious diseases

Hypothermia   a condition in which the central body temperature drops below 35°C

Immune system   fights infections (caused by germs) using white cells in the blood, including lymphocytes

Immunisation   the process of strengthening the immune system often with a vaccine

Immunity   a protection against infectious diseases

Incontinence   loss of voluntary control of the bladder or bowels

Infectious disease   illness caused by germs that spread from one person to another

Interpersonal skills   the skills used when people communicate with each other including the ability to relate to other people. *See* **Communication**

Labelling   a short-cut, and often inaccurate, way of describing or classifying people in a word or phrase

Legislation   the making of laws and regulations by parliament

Leukaemia   a type of cancer in the bone marrow that results in too many, and abnormal, white cells in the blood

Lifestyle   the way in which a person chooses to live their life

Loneliness   being cut-off from contact with other people

Malnutrition   a condition caused by too much food, insufficient food, or an unbalanced diet. It can lead to obesity, starvation, or deficiency diseases

Media   'mass media' includes television, radio, newspapers, magazines and mass advertisements

Meningitis   inflammation of the membranes covering the brain and spinal cord

Organ   a part of the body with a special function or functions

Palliative care   a support system to help ease the many problems of people who are terminally ill, and their families

Paralysis   loss of muscle power in a part of the body, usually caused by a stroke or nerve injury

Paraplegia   paralysis of the lower half of the body due to damage of the spinal cord

Pharmacist   a person with a degree in pharmacy who is qualified to dispense medicines and give advice on their use

Physiology   how the body works

Plaque   a gooey substance. In the arteries, it consists mainly of cholesterol and can build up to block the artery. *See* **Atheroma**. In the mouth, it is a different gooey substance that builds up between the teeth

Plasma   the pale yellow liquid in which the blood cells are suspended

Political factors   those relating to government policies and legislation

Posture   the way the body is held when standing, sitting, walking, bending or lifting

Poverty   absolute poverty is not having enough money to pay for items essential to life. Relative poverty is not having the goods, services and pleasures that other people take for granted

Prejudice   judging people before knowing enough about them

Pressure sores   Skin ulcers on the 'pressure areas' (buttocks, heels, elbows) of patients confined to bed. *See* **Bedsores**

Pro-social behaviour   behaviour that involves others with sharing, helping and caring. *See* **Anti-social behaviour**

Psychiatrist   a doctor who specialises in the study and treatment of mental disorders

Psychologist   a person with a degree in psychology. A Clinical Psychologist has a higher degree in psychology

Psychology   the study of the mind: normal and abnormal behaviour

Pulse   a wave of blood that is pumped through the arteries with each heartbeat. It can be felt where an artery lies over hard tissue and just under the skin

Quadriplegia   paralysis of all four limbs due to damage to the spinal cord in the neck

Rash   an outbreak of red spots or patches on the skin

Records   keeping information about what has occurred

Rehabilitation   restoration of or moving towards normal function

Relationships   personal links with other people

Relaxation   a result of reduced mental and physical pressure

Religion   belief in and worship of an all-powerful supernatural power, God

Respite care   provides a break from a too-demanding daily routine for clients and their carers

Risk   the likelihood that a hazard will cause harm. *See* **Hazard**

Self-concept   'who you think you are' – a combination of self-esteem and self-image

Self-esteem   how you value yourself as a person

Self-image   your internal picture of yourself – what you look like and how you behave

Serum   the fluid that seeps out of blood clots. It is plasma without the clotting factors

Service providers   organisations that provide caring services (e.g., hospitals and health centres)

Service users   patients, clients or customers who use the health and social care services (e.g., patients use health care services, clients or customers use social care services)

Sexuality   the way people express the sexual aspects of their lives. It is often used to mean sexual orientation (homosexual, heterosexual, etc.)

Social care   support for people who need help to meet their personal and social needs, but not their medical needs

Social class   a group of people who share a common position in society

Social exclusion   being unable to access the things in life that most people take for granted

Social Services   provide welfare services for people at times when they need care and support

Socialisation   learning to become part of a social group: social development

Social worker   a degree-qualified professional who helps people with personal, emotional or financial problems

Society   a group of individuals living together in an organised way with common characteristics such as nationality, race or religion

Socio-economic factors   people- and money-related factors such as income, housing, education, and life-style activities

Statutory service   a service, e.g. the NHS and Social Services, provided by government statutes (laws)

Stereotyping   putting people into groups based on features that they are assumed to have in common

Stress   emotional or mental tension or strain produced by too much or prolonged pressure

Stroke   the weakness or paralysis (often down one side) that occurs when the normal blood supply to a part of the brain is cut off

Substance abuse   the misuse of substances such as drugs, solvents and alcohol

Sympathy   understanding someone else's situation. *See* **Empathy**

System   a group of organs in the body that work together to carry out one or more functions

Terminal illness   an illness that will end in death, often within a clearly limited time

Therapeutic activities   aim to improve health and mobility

Therapy   treatment

Tinnitus   ringing, buzzing or whistling sounds in the ear, sometimes interfering with hearing

Tissue   a group of cells specialised to perform a particular function

Ulcer   a break in any surface inside or outside the body that fails to heal or heals only slowly

Vaccination   the administration of a vaccine to produce immunity to a disease

Varicose veins   swollen veins usually seen on the legs

Vein   returns blood back to the heart

Victimisation   singling somebody out (the victim) for hostile or unfair treatment

Virus (plural, viruses)   a group of microbes even smaller than bacteria. *See* **Bacteria**

Vitamin   a substance essential for the normal functioning of the body, needed in only a very small quantity

Vulnerable   people who are easily hurt and have poor defences

Wellbeing   a feeling of control over life with optimism about the future

WHO   World Health Organization

Work experience   time in a place of work learning about a particular job or area of work

Index (Page numbers in **bold** indicate the main reference for an item.)